FUNDAMENTALS
OF PRIVATE PRACTICE
IN PHYSICAL THERAPY

FUNDAMENTALS OF PRIVATE PRACTICE IN PHYSICAL THERAPY

By

MARK A. BRIMER, P.T., M.B.A.

Illustrations and Photography by

John F. Braun

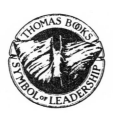

CHARLES C THOMAS • PUBLISHER
Springfield • Illinois • U.S.A.

Published and Distributed Throughout the World by

CHARLES C THOMAS • PUBLISHER

2600 South First Street

Springfield, Illinois 62794-9265

© *1988 by* CHARLES C THOMAS • PUBLISHER

ISBN 0-398-05448-7

Library of Congress Catalog Card Number: 87-37451

With THOMAS BOOKS *careful attention is given to all details of manufacturing and design. It is the Publisher's desire to present books that are satisfactory as to their physical qualities and artistic possibilities and appropriate for their particular use.* THOMAS BOOKS *will be true to those laws of quality that assure a good name and good will.*

Printed in the United States of America

Q-R-3

Library of Congress Cataloging in Publication Data

Brimer, Mark A.
    Fundamentals of private practice in physical therapy.

    Includes index.
    1. Physical therapy--Practice. I. Title.
[DNLM: 1. Physical Therapy. 2. Private Practice--
organization & administration. WB 460 B857f]
RM705.B75   1988   362.1'78   87-37451
ISBN 0-398-05448-7

To my wife, Leslee,
my parents,
and sons, Eric and Christopher

INTRODUCTION

THE PRACTICE of physical therapy in the United States is presently in a state of evolution. Increasing numbers of physical therapists are establishing private practice facilities or are seriously considering the sometimes difficult task of establishing an individual or group practice in physical therapy.

The opportune time to establish a private practice in physical therapy is approaching. By the year 2000 there will be more than thirty-three million Americans over the age of sixty-five. Approximately one in every eight U.S. citizens will be in that age group. As the average age of the population continues to rise, an increasing number of individuals will, at some period in their life, require physical therapy.

Good business management is essential to a good physical therapy practice. A private practitioner who ignores the basic principles of business is likely to find it impossible to meet salary needs and expenses.

Patients, due in part to the high cost of today's medical care, are increasingly dependent on third-party programs or insurance to help offset their costs. It is essential that each patient have well-documented and properly prepared records to enable their claims to be processed quickly. Inefficient systems of patient billing and record keeping frequently slow down the process of payment to the private practitioner. Haphazard office procedures may also raise a question in the patient's mind as to whether a physical therapist with a poorly run office is competent to make quality decisions regarding the provision of health care.

Many physical therapists are turning to proven management methods and techniques which can be easily adapted to a private practice setting. For example, the ease of use of the modern computer can greatly reduce the time and complexity involved in patient billing. Other methods are also available to assist the practitioner in the proper recruitment and selection of office personnel.

As a result of the constantly changing environment of the health care provider, the daily operation of a private practice is becoming more difficult. There are several areas of business a practitioner must fully understand in order to operate a successful practice. These are: basic accounting and finance, professional and personal liability insurance, real estate, medical record keeping, and personnel management.

Good management techniques applied to a private practice in physical therapy are not unprofessional. There is a business side to any medical practice. The therapist who applies proper management techniques will be able to spend more time with patients or pursue leisure activities.

This book examines the basic management principles available to the physical therapist to assist in the planning, financing, design, and operation of a private practice, physical therapy center. It is designed for the physical therapist who is contemplating the opening of an outpatient facility or for the established practitioner to use as a tool to evaluate effectiveness and efficiency. It should afford the reader the most modern techniques to ensure the proper set up and management of a private practice at the lowest possible cost.

CONTENTS

FUNDAMENTALS
OF PRIVATE PRACTICE
IN PHYSICAL THERAPY

CHAPTER ONE

WHERE TO BEGIN

FOR MANY physical therapists, the most difficult step in opening a private practice is to determine where to begin. The process of opening a practice by yourself can be very long, frustrating, and expensive if you are starting with a limited business background. Should you begin by locating professional office space? Is it best to start with an examination of your financial position? These are important questions, but do not constitute the best starting position.

The first step in opening a private practice is to determine what type of practice you would like to have. There are three basic practice options available. The first is to look into becoming an associate with an already established practitioner who is in need of an additional therapist. Frequently, a practitioner makes this opportunity available in an effort to lessen the patient load currently being carried by the individual member. Another option is to open your own office by yourself or with one or more partners. The third option is to contract for your services. This is generally done with a hospital or nursing home facility.

PRIVATE PRACTITIONER AS AN ASSOCIATE WITH AN ESTABLISHED PRACTITIONER

One of the least expensive methods to become a private practice physical therapist is to become an associate with a practitioner in an established office. Under this arrangement you may eventually enter into a partnership agreement allowing you a portion of the profits. The agreement you sign will stipulate the period of time (generally several months to years) before you become a partner. Your portion of the profits is dependent upon the terms of the agreement.

An associate practice can be personally and financially rewarding depending on the location, personalities involved, and the terms of the agreement. Practices such as these may also develop from the discussions students have while in school. Each student hopes to someday open a practice as a joint venture.

Occasionally, difficulties in associate relationships may arise. These can be avoided by carefully worded contracts between the parties which spell out the areas of extreme importance. In most instances, it is better to have a trial period to see if both parties can comfortably work together. The trial period may last months to years.

FLORIDA

Private Practice

Full time Florida licensed or eligible. Opportunity for junior partnership. East Central Florida. Excellent salary plus benefits. Send resume or call. Box xx Anytown, FL 00000 305/000/0000

Figure I. Ads such as these frequently appear in professional journals and magazines. It is advisable to first telephone the practitioner and discuss the practice situation before sending the resume.

In private practice situations such as these you will generally be hired first as an employee. Your salary is often determined by how much your services are needed and how close your working relationship will be. If, after the trial period, the relationship appears to be working well you may be promoted to an associate position. This will allow your compensation to be adjusted to a level that more closely reflects the actual contribution that you, as an individual, are making to the overall practice.

In some private practice situations you may be offered the opportunity to buy into the practice gradually. This may be done over a period of years to a point where you reach equal participation with the other associates in the practice.

In either practice opportunity have the proposed written agreement reviewed by an attorney. Make sure the agreement spells out the appropriate timetable and methods of payment. Do not rely solely on a handshake. It is recommended that you avoid the contribution of any money until you have had the opportunity to evaluate the personnel you will be working with as well as the local community.

OPENING AN INDIVIDUAL PRACTICE

To open an individual office is the ideal situation for most physical therapists. For many therapists, the individual office may be the most difficult, but is generally the most professionally rewarding. In a situation such as this, the practitioner has total responsibility for all aspects of the practice. It often requires a maximum expenditure of time to develop the private office into a successful practice.

As an individual owner of the practice, you must frequently donate a large percentage of your free time to community-related activities. These activities will allow you to associate with others who will be essential in referring patients to your practice. Depending on the location of your practice and the availability of similar practices, it may take several months before your practice becomes profitable.

As more therapists establish private practices, there will be increasing opportunities to purchase an existing private practice. These opportunities will arise as an individual practitioner reaches retirement age and desires to sell the practice. Such opportunities as these can eliminate the long wait for a patient load to be established. It is important, however, that proper valuation techniques be applied to judge the actual dollar value of the practice. Many factors must be considered before determining the potential of an ongoing practice. Financial disaster can occur if a practice is purchased with a large number of unpaid patient bills which have little chance of ever being collected.

FLORIDA

Private Practice for Sale

2400 Sq. Ft. office with 50-60 patient per day capacity, ocean view. Full compliment of weight equipment and rehab modalities. Assume lease and accounts receivable.   305/XXX/XXXX

Pediatric private practice for sale. Located in Southeast, specializing in the treatment of Cerebral Palsy and Down's syndrome. Complete, well-trained staff with up-to-date equipment.
305/000/0000

Figure II. Ads such as these tell you little about the practice. Both practices sound like excellent opportunities but will need to be thoroughly examined to ascertain their overall potential.

CONTRACTING FOR YOUR SERVICES

A large number of physical therapists begin a private practice through a contract with another party. Generally these contracts are with nursing homes, school districts, home health agencies, or hospitals. These forms of private practice are very popular in areas where the shortage of physical therapists is severe. Once established, they can lead to excellent opportunities to open individual offices.

When contracting for services it is essential that both parties involved have a clear written agreement as to the method of payment to be made to the contracting physical therapist. Generally, the therapist should be paid at least monthly by the contracting facility.

When negotiating with a facility, be realistic. In some instances, physical therapists have successfully submitted the lowest bid to provide services only to find the volume of work required far exceeds the compensation provided. Know exactly what you are getting into before signing a contract which you may not be able to fulfill.

SHOULD I INCORPORATE?

A corporation is a legal entity completely separate and apart from its members. It is one of the most prevalent forms of business organization in the United States.

There are many benefits as well as drawbacks to the incorporation of a private practice in physical therapy. Many physical therapists avoid forming a corporation because they believe it will be too complicated or take too much time away from patients or their family to operate the practice properly. Depending upon the practice, the decision not to incorporate may cost the practitioner thousands of dollars in additional tax payments.

In most states, corporate forms of medical practice are referred to as professional associations (P.A.), professional corporations (P.C.), or service corporations (S.C.). Virtually all states have a "Professional Associations Act" which allows the practice of professionals (therapists, doctors, dentists, and lawyers) under the corporate form. The primary objective of the Professional Associations Act is to allow a professional to obtain tax advantages not available to individuals or partnerships.

Practically every state incorporation statue requires that no professional corporation name will be the same as or similar to the name of any existing corporation in the same state. Many physical therapists avoid problems such as these by using either their last name or the name of the town in which the practice is located.

Once formed, the corporation becomes an independent tax-paying business which is completely separate from you or any other physical therapists who are also shareholders in the corporation. Income and expenses of the corporation are kept separate from any personal finances. The corporation must abide by state and federal laws as well as tax obligations. The corporation is considered separate from the practitioner even if the practitioner is the only stockholder in the corporation.

In the nonmedical business community one of the attractive aspects of incorporation as compared to the development of a partnership is the concept of limited liability. Limited liability provides that an individual shareholder (a person owning stock in the company) is only liable for the contracts and debts up to the dollar value of the corporations stock that they own.

Professional corporations do not have the provisions for limited liability. In a professional corporation, in which the shareholders are physical therapists, they retain their unlimited liability for injuries to the patients they treat. Therefore, the decision to incorporate to lessen the individual therapist's liability should not be the primary reason for the incorporation of a private practice.

In some states the decision whether or not to incorporate may help limit your liability in the event of a malpractice claim. If a fellow shareholder commits a medical malpractice, it is possible you may be only held liable up to the amount you have invested in the corporation. In a partnership, the malpractice judgement would first be paid by the insurance company (up to the limit of the policy) then by the partnership assets, then by the individual therapist, and finally by any or all of the remaining partners. In a partnership, each partner is responsible for the actions of the others.

Incorporation also limits the liability for acts by employees to the assets of the corporation. Depending upon the state, if an employee commits an act of negligence and you are not incorporated, the damages would first be paid up to the limit of the insurance policy, then by the business assets, then out of your own personal assets.

One of the most attractive aspects of a corporate form of physical therapy practice is the advantages of reduced state and federal taxes. Other advantages include employee benefit programs and investments. A corporation may make deposits into pensions and employee profit sharing programs. These deposits can be deducted from the corporation's taxable income. The funds are held until a future date when they can be paid out to the employees. The interest earned on these funds is added to the programs on a tax free basis.

Group insurance may also be available to the physical therapist in a professional corporation. Group insurance is one of the oldest and most common benefits to employees. It generally includes health, life and disability. Under group insurance the insurance company generally makes no selection of the individuals it will insure. The insurance company sets the premiums according to the characteristics of the group as a whole. Many insurance companies require a certain number of people as an employed group before providing coverage. This is to avoid adverse risks and lower administrative costs. Group term life insurance is generally offered without a physical examination and has no loan provisions, cash surrender value or paid up value.

There are some disadvantages to incorporation. Once incorporated you will be spending more time with paper work. Incorporation forces the management of all financial records. Because of this you may need the assistance of a certified public accountant (C.P.A.) to manage all of your financial obligations.

The final decision to incorporate must be based upon the perceived advantages and disadvantages of incorporation. In order to properly incorporate a practice carefully select an attorney with a proven record in establishing professional corporations.

CONTRACTS

Depending upon the type of practice arrangement you are developing, either a partnership or a corporation, you will be asked to enter into some form of written agreement. This agreement is solely to protect the personal and financial interests of all parties involved.

When presented with a contract it is always best to consult an attorney prior to signing the contract. The contract you are considering should be clearly worded so each party knows exactly what to expect of the other.

The most important items to consider in any professional contract are as follows:

1. The name of the organization with an indication as to whether it is a partnership or a corporation.

2. A description of the type of services to be performed. An example: The purpose of the partnership is to engage in the business of providing physical therapy services to the public for profit.

3. The principle place of business. A listing of the street address, city, and state are all that are required.

4. Initial capital contributions. Capital refers to resources invested (money, equipment) in a firm by creditors and owners. It should also be indicated if future additional capital contributions will be required.

5. The length of time each member is to remain on salary. Depending on the prospective arrangement you may be able to negotiate a shorter period than is initially proposed.

6. Duties and rights of all partners.

7. The conditions under which you will become a partner, associate or shareholder.

8. Provisions for reimbursement of travel, educational and entertainment expenses.

9. The methods of bookkeeping.

10. The length of the agreement as well as how it can be terminated.

11. The determination of a bank account and the distribution of funds.

12. Substitutions, assignments, and admissions of additional partners.

13. The return of capital contributions upon dissolution of the partnership or corporation.

14. Payment for interest of a deceased general partner. This allows your spouse to receive the funds you would have been entitled to before your death.

15. Provisions for amendments. This usually indicates how the signed agreement can be modified.

16. Additional purchase options. This may allow you to purchase additional interest in the practice at a future date.

17. Noncompetition covenant. These convenants are used to protect the senior partner in a practice who has spent a great deal of time and money recruiting an associate. If after a period of time the new partner decides to leave the practice and locate a new practice in the same locale, the senior partner may suffer economic losses due to a loss of business. To prevent this, most contracts between professionals provide that in the event that you are unable to perform, or cease to perform services for the practice, you will not either directly or indirectly become involved in another practice for a specified number of years within a certain distance. Many contracts specify the period and distance to be three years and fifteen miles. Keep in mind, noncompetition covenants are legally enforceable and persons violating these covenants may be sued to prevent further violation and to collect economic damages as a result of their actions.

DETERMINATION OF A LOCATION: THE MAJOR FACTORS TO CONSIDER

Once you have decided the type of practice you would like to establish, the next critical step in the process of setting up a private practice is the determination of a location. This step may indeed be the most crucial. An error in the selection of a practice location could result in a great deal of financial difficulty. A prolonged period of time without patients could result in personal frustrations to you and your family.

One of the safest ways to determine a location in which to establish a practice is to work in a community where you believe there lies the greatest number of opportunities. Many physical therapists begin private practices in this manner. They simply choose a hospital setting and survey the community and the type of patients which arrive for treatment. After several years of employment they generally have accumulated sufficient funds and have enough confidence in the community's potential to go out on their own.

Setting up a practice in this manner has been quite successful for many physical therapists. This will also work very well in regions of the country where private practice in physical therapy is not yet well established. As competition increases you will need to use additional criteria to evaluate a community. The following four areas of analysis are becoming more important as competition for the health care dollar continues.

ECONOMIC ANALYSIS

The analysis of a community's economy need not be a difficult process. There are a number of observable factors which make up a local economy. The level of industrialization and measurements of population growth or decline are some of the factors which can be easily analyzed.

The best way to begin your economic analysis of a community is to simply drive down many of the city streets that are within a five to ten mile radius of your proposed location. An examination of the type of housing available in the community as well as the occupancy rates can tell you if an area is growing, holding its own, or on the downslide.

Population is another way to determine practice potential. Contact the local chamber of commerce to obtain information on which areas of the community are growing, by what percent a year, and what most of these people do for a living. Many orthopaedic surgeons feel they can make a comfortable living with a ratio of one surgeon per every twenty thousand people. Check the local yellow pages and determine the number of private clinics and divide that number into the population. Depending on your therapy speciality this may be one simple method to determine relative need.

In many cases the physicians in a community can provide information about a community's potential. They are in constant contact with local real estate agents, bankers, and business people. Physicians can supply information about the strengths and weaknesses of the local medical staff. Check with the medical staff office in the local hospital. All physicians applying for staff privileges must submit their applications through that office. The secretary in the office can inform you whether staff membership is increasing. If it is increasing, try to determine by how much and in what specialities.

Even more information can be obtained by talking with the therapists in the hospital's physical therapy department. Find out if the area is in need of additional therapists. Ask their opinion of the local community.

GEOGRAPHICAL
AND ENVIRONMENTAL ANALYSIS

There are many factors which may be considered as making up the geography and environment of an area. The first step is to analyze the local community to see if it is subject to seasonal fluctuations. For example, in some parts of Florida, a community may see a great influx of elderly people during the winter months. Many of the elderly come to their winter home during the months of November thru March to avoid the bitter northern cold. During this same period of time many Florida hospitals experience a rise in their census due to an increase in elective surgery. A physical therapy private practice may do extremely well during the winter months but experience slow periods in the summer. A physical therapist who opens a practice at the end of March could have a financially difficult time of surviving the summer.

Industrial expansion is also a good indicator of private practice potential. Industries which recruit high tech people such as computer scientists and engineers frequently pay their people well above the national average and provide a wide assortment of benefits. Talk with people familiar with these industries. They can be of help in locating regions of the country where the corporate leaders of technology and computer development are locating. Towns in which major segments of an industry are closing would not be areas to invest your valuable time and money.

Attempt to determine if the tax delinquency rate for an area is rising. People who are unable to pay their taxes would also be unlikely to pay their physical therapy bills. The county tax collector's office should be able to provide this information.

Determine where most patients go for their outpatient physical therapy. What factors influence their decision to choose that facility? Local physicians will tell you whether the current facility meets their needs and how you could better serve the community.

Visit one of the larger banks in the community. Ask about the economy of the area. Are bank deposits increasing or decreasing? Has there been an increase in the number of new mortgages or mortgage foreclosures? Inform the bank representative of your plans and ask for an opinion as to its potential in the community.

PROFESSIONAL ANALYSIS

Your background, experience, and professional aspirations have a great deal to do with how you will approach a private practice. If you are the type of physical therapist who feels uncomfortable without the availability of the latest diagnostic aids and modern facilities close at hand you may find it difficult to make the adjustment to practicing individually in a small community. It is however, important that you not completely overlook these areas since the local hospital may be heavily recruiting talented physicians and medical personnel to fill the void. In general, it is best to eliminate those areas where you most definitely would not want to establish a private practice. Then your chances of choosing the right location will be better wherever you go.

After your search has determined several specific communities of interest, you should make a thorough examination of all available medical facilities. If you intend to go into a solo practice you will need to examine what sort of office space is available. Location of the office is, of course, the most important factor. Generally, the closer the office is to hospitals and other medical offices the better. The site under consideration should have ample parking and ease of accessibility. If you are considering an association with another physical therapist you should carefully examine their office facilities as well as the age and type of equipment being utilized.

Talk with the hospital administrator. He/she can provide you with additional information about the medical staff. Ask whether the hospital has any plans for expansion. If the hospital does have plans for expansion it will give you some clue as to the potential growth of the community. The hospital, which requires a certificate of need for expansion, would only attempt an expansion if there is a good expectation of community growth.

Examine the services available in the community which could be used to assist your practice. Is there a good medical supply company which will sell walkers, canes, and crutches? What services are available to amputees? Do the elderly have a transportation system which could be utilized at your proposed location? Determine the opportunities for professional growth. Is there an active physical therapy study group, or will you suffer professional isolation if you settle in the area?

Evaluate the local nursing home facilities. Are most of the nursing homes medicare/medicaid or are they private pay? Talk with several nursing home administrators and find out how much they utilize physical therapy. Ask to see the physical therapy department and equipment available for patient treatment.

PERSONAL EXPECTATIONS

You must determine whether the community you are evaluating is a good place to live. You need to examine that aspect from your own perspective as well as from your family's point of view. Depending on your previous life style you will have to adjust your social activities to fit with what the community has to offer. Fitting into the community is essential to the survival of your practice.

In the beginning you will be putting in long hours to develop your practice. It is very important to involve your spouse in the choice of a community in which to establish a practice. Both you and your spouse should examine the social, religious, educational, and recreational opportunities in the community. It is essential that they meet your needs.

What type of schooling is available to the children in the community? Will they have to ride buses to school? Are day care centers and shopping centers easily accessible? No community will offer everything you would like to have. It is important to determine whether the community will, over the years, continue to offer the opportunity to make a reasonable living and afford you and your family with personal satisfaction.

CHAPTER TWO

THE FINANCIAL ASPECTS OF PRACTICE

THERE IS never a perfect time to open a private practice. No matter how much you plan there will always be an element of financial risk. You can lessen the risk and increase the probability of success if you carefully examine your professional goals and your financial position.

To properly calculate the cost of starting and operating a private practice requires that you become acquainted with terminology common to the business environment. Understanding business terminology will allow you to identify problem areas in practice. Once problems are identified, you are better able to make decisions about the necessity of contacting professionals to assist in correcting the problem.

The following sections will provide information with which the practitioner must be familiar in order to survive in the competitive health care environment. Quite often, the one thing that prevents many physical therapists from starting their own practice is money. They feel it will either be too expensive to start a practice or too risky to gamble on the potential success of a practice. This chapter discusses the money needed to own and operate a practice, and how to invest it wisely.

ANALYZING FINANCIAL OPPORTUNITIES FOR PRACTICE

There are a great number of risks involved in the opening of a private practice. It is often difficult to determine how much to spend on office space and medical equipment while still having enough money left over to pay employee salaries and meeting your own living expenses.

The majority of physical therapists like medical doctors, dentists, and lawyers are not financially prepared to start out building or buying an office. Financially, in many cases, the best approach is to practice in a community for at least six months to one year before investing in the acquisition of commercial buildings or real estate. There are, however, a number of ways to establish a practice. Each has advantages and disadvantages.

When evaluating office space, the most important consideration is the floor plan. The practice should be designed so it will allow the most efficient use of employee time in patient treatment. The exact space requirements for a practice will depend on the scope of the physical therapy services to be provided. The minimum space requirements for the beginning practitioner will range from eight hundred to one thousand square feet up to a maximum of fifteen hundred to sixteen hundred square feet.

In the process of evaluating an office space, give careful consideration to the future expansion plans of the practice. As the practice grows you will want to add employees and provide greater services. The evaluation of a proposed location should include expansion plans for a larger waiting room, receptionists area, and storage space for patient records.

The decision of where to locate a practice may be crucial to its financial survival. Very often the location will determine how rapidly a practice will grow. Many practitioners choose to locate in a medical office building. The rationale behind this practice location is the belief the practice obtains an advantage because it is exposed to patients already accustomed to visiting the medical center. Physicians own a large percentage of medical offices. When designing medical offices, physicians try to meet the needs of fellow medical professionals. Some medical buildings therefore require less renovation before starting a practice than nonmedical offices.

The lease price for office space is most heavily influenced by its location in a community. It may cost anywhere from eight to ten dollars per square foot in newer medical office buildings. Older buildings may have per square foot costs of six to seven dollars. More expensive or "prime locations" may run as high as thirty dollars per square foot.

If you decide that a private practice would best be located in a nonmedical building, assess the surrounding community in which the practice would be located. Is the prospective building, or any other nearby structure, deteriorating? Does the building's owner have any plans to renovate the structure? A practice located in a small shopping center may do well if the community is growing.

Evaluate each prospective location in terms of its accessibility. The easier it is to get to your practice, the more likely patients are to seek out your services. Will the practice remain that way? Practitioners have located below market prices for office space only to discover that extensive road construction is planned which would make patient access to the facility difficult. Check with the city road department director about plans for road improvements or construction.

Practitioners often investigate the financial investment required to remodel an existing office or residence. Remodeling can be very expensive. Many of the financial costs must be borne by the practitioner, since few landlords will provide assistance. Most leases provide that any remodeling done will accrue to the building's owner. It is best to keep remodeling to a minimum unless you plan to be in the location for a long period of time or can obtain a long-term lease.

New practitioners should consider the use of curtains and moveable particians to wall off areas of patient treatment. The construction of permanent walls may require building code approval. As the practice grows, curtains and moveable particians provide greater flexibility in rearranging the office.

If the proposed office must be remodeled, have the structure examined by a professional real estate appraiser or architect. Determine the adequacy and age of the heating and air conditioning, electrical system, and plumbing. Physical therapy must allow for a large usage of electricity to safely operate all medical equipment. Electrical grounding, sometimes not up to code requirements in older buildings, is especially important. The plumbing should be sufficient to allow for quick filling and drainage of whirlpools. The water heater should be large enough to heat a great volume of water as quickly as possible. A physical therapy department can use several hundred gallons of heated water per hour. Improper water heater size could limit your practice's ability to adequately meet patient needs.

When reviewing a location for its potential, do not let others talk you into an inconvenient location or a poor floor plan. Try to lease enough space which will allow the practice to grow without becoming overwhelmed with large lease payments.

IF YOU DECIDE TO LEASE

After careful examination of all options you may decide that leasing office space will provide the best practice opportunity. When presented with a lease, read it very carefully. Do not sign it without a thorough understanding of each clause contained in the lease. If necessary, review the lease with an attorney to clarify any questions you may have.

A lease should contain a complete description of the building to be leased. Included should be a description of the conditions of each room and any furnishings which are provided. The lease should also specify what services are to be provided by the building's owner. Some indication should be made as to who will pay for restoration of the building once you vacate the premises.

The lease should allow you to sublet the premises in the event you are no longer able to practice at the location. A provision should also be made which will allow the termination of the lease with a full return of the deposit. Make sure there is a description of the insurance required to adequately protect the building. A provision should also be made which will let you out of the lease if there is damage which renders the building unfit for occupancy.

Try to negotiate a lease which will provide the building rent free for the first few months of occupancy. In some areas there may be an abundance of rental property available. The owner may be anxious to rent the property and forgo the first few months of rent if you will agree to a long-term lease. In other cases, the owner will allow the rent to be paid at a later date, once the practice is established. The initial savings can be very helpful to getting a practice started.

LEASING OFFICE SPACE

Advantages:

1. Leasing provides flexibility. If you find the location undesirable, you can move at the end of the lease.
2. The buildings' maintenance is the landlord's responsibility.
3. Minimal time is needed before the building can be occupied.
4. In many cases, the owner of the building will provide personnel for cleaning the office.

Disadvantages:

1. Leasing does not provide a build up of equity.
2. You have little control over the maintenance of the building.
3. Tax deductions cannot be made for building depreciation.
4. Rent generally increases at lease-renewal time.
5. Improvements made to the building, such as the addition of cabinets and plumbing installation often accrue to the owner.

RENOVATING A BUILDING

Advantages:

1. Depending on the location, the cost may be very reasonable.
2. The building can be depreciated for tax purposes.
3. In many cases, landscaping has already been done.

Disadvantages:

1. The floor plan may be unsuitable.
2. The building may be poorly insulated.
3. Existing plumbing and electrical outlets may need replacement.
4. Maintenance costs on the building's exterior may be higher than new construction.

BUILDING OR BUYING AN OFFICE

Advantages:

1. The building can be designed according to your needs.
2. There is a build up of equity in the mortgage.
3. The building can be depreciated for tax purposes.
4. There is no obligation to a landlord.

Disadvantages:

1. Building or buying an office can be very expensive.
2. It may be difficult to sell the office.
3. Construction costs are high.
4. Maintenance is your responsibility.
5. Expansion may be required due to practice growth.

Figure III. Buy, build, or lease? There are a number of things to consider before making the financial investment.

UNDERSTANDING FINANCIAL STATEMENTS

The ability to communicate with those individuals who will assess the financial health of the practice is essential. Accountants and tax attorneys will provide investment guidance based on their assessment of the financial performance of the practice. For the practitioner, the two most important financial statements are the balance sheet and the income statement. Understanding these areas of business is essential to a working knowledge of the bookkeeping necessary to operate a private practice.

THE BALANCE SHEET

The balance sheet is a financial statement that indicates the financial performance of the practice on a specific date. Accountants usually prepare a balance sheet for the date that marks the end of the year for the practice. For most practices, the date that represents the end of the year is December 31. It is important to realize, however, that a balance sheet can be developed for any date. Some businesses develop them quarterly, semiannually, as well as annually.

The balance sheet is divided into two parts; the assets owed by the practice and the claims made against these assets by creditors. The claims made by creditors are called liabilities. The remaining interest in the practice, listed on the same side as the liabilities, is called owners equity. The basic format of the balance sheet separates assets from the liabilities and the owners equity.

BALANCE SHEET FOR ANYTOWN P.T.

Assets	Liabilities & Owners Equity

Figure IV.

Assets are, in most cases, tangible items such as cash, land, buildings, or equipment. They are visible and easily identified as part of the therapy practice. Assets can, however, be tangible. Examples of intangible assets are patents and copyrights. Although not visible, they can have a value to the practice of several thousand dollars.

Liabilities are the debts of the practice. Examples of liabilities include outstanding loans, electric bills, and mortgage payments. Liabilities can be divided into two categories; either short-term liabilities (sometimes called current liabilities) or long-term liabilities. Short-term liabilities are those debts due within the year. Long-term liabilities are due in the future, usually longer than one year away. Long-term loans are most often made for building mortgages or land purchases.

Owner's equity is the remaining amount after the practice debts have been subtracted from the practice assets. The owner's equity will increase when the practice is making money and decline when the practice suffers a financial loss.

EXAMINING THE BALANCE SHEET

To understand how the balance sheet is utilized in the business environment of the practice, it is necessary to analyze a simplified version of an actual balance sheet. Figure V provides an example of Anytown Physical Therapy's balance sheet dated December 31, 19XX. Included are the three areas present on all balance sheets; the assets, liabilities, and the owner's equity.

The following terms highlight the importance to the practitioner of identifying and understanding each account on the balance sheet.

Current Assets. Current assets are cash and other items that are expected to be converted to cash or consumed during a normal, one-year operating cycle.

Cash. Cash consists of any currency, checks, or bank account balances belonging to the practice.

Accounts Receivable. Accounts receivable is a current asset which represents claims against patients for unpaid services. The services include all treatments performed by the practice.

Allowance for Uncollectables. Not all patients will pay for the services they received from the practice. Allowance for uncollectables indicates the amount of receivables that are expected to be uncollectable. In health care, as much as ten percent or more may be uncollectable. Tightening credit standards will help reduce uncollectable accounts.

BALANCE SHEET				
	ASSETS	Anytown Physical Therapy December 31, 19XX	LIABILITIES	
CURRENT ASSETS			**CURRENT LIABILITIES**	
Cash		10,000	Accounts Payable	1,500
Accounts Receivable	45,000		Taxes Payable	12,500
Less: Allowance for uncollectable accounts	5,000	40,000	Loan Payable	11,000
Prepaid Expenses		2,000	**TOTAL CURRENT LIABILITIES**	$ 25,000
TOTAL CURRENT ASSETS		$ 52,000	**LONG TERM LIABILITIES**	
FIXED ASSETS			Bank Loan	$115,000
Land		75,000	**TOTAL LIABILITIES**	$140,000
Building	125,000			
Less Depreciation	25,000	100,000	**OWNER'S EQUITY**	
Equipment	50,000		Total Owner's Equity	$27,000
Less Depreciation	10,000	40,000		
TOTAL FIXED ASSETS		$115,000		
TOTAL ASSETS		$167,000	**TOTAL LIABILITIES AND OWNERS EQUITY**	$167,000

Figure V.

Prepaid Expenses. This asset is an expense, such as insurance, which has been paid but not entirely utilized. Many insurance policies are paid either semiannually or annually. They must be carried as an asset until consumed.

Fixed Assets. Assets such as land, buildings, machinery, equipment, are considered fixed assets. A fixed asset will be held by the practice for an extended period of time, usually several years.

Land. Land is recorded on the balance sheet at its full cost. Periodically the value of the land may be increased on the balance sheet to reflect its actual resale value.

Buildings. This is the location of the practice. If the practice has two locations, both are listed.

Accumulated Depreciation on the Building. A term used primarily for tax purposes, depreciation indicates the amount of the original price of the building which has been subtracted due to wear and obsolence. Depreciation reduces the amount of taxable income and helps lower tax liability.

Equipment. This asset includes all machinery and office furniture belonging to the practice. For tax purposes, equipment is also shown at its depreciated value.

Current Liabilities. Current liabilities are debts owed by the practice which must be paid during the next year or within the practice's normal operating cycle.

Accounts Payable. This account represents debts owed by the practice for services or goods purchased on credit. Examples include repairs made by service technicians on practice equipment which have an outstanding amount due to the company who provided the repair service.

Taxes Payable. Taxes payable represent money owed to the federal, state, or local government. Practitioners may be required to pay income taxes on a quarterly basis.

Loan Payable. Listed under current liabilities, loan payable represents the amount due in the coming year. The remainder of the debt is carried as a long-term liability.

Long-Term Liability. In many practice situations, long-term debts are bank loans. They will not be due during the current operating cycle. As seen from Figure V, $11,000 of the loan will be paid during this year. The remaining $115,000 will be paid over the next several years.

Owner's Equity. Owner's equity refers to the total assets of the practice not claimed by the creditors. Sometimes referred to as "net worth" or "net assets," it represents total assets minus total liabilities.

THE INCOME STATEMENT

The income statement is a financial statement that shows changes that have occurred in the practice over a period of time. For accounting purposes, the period of time is generally one year. This is in contrast to the balance sheet which reflects the financial position of the practice on a specific date. The income statement, for example, will show changes in the financial position of the practice for this year in comparison to last year.

When an accountant prepares the practice income statement, it will report the financial success (or failure) of the practice during the period of time under examination. The statement will identify whether revenues were greater (or less) than expenses. In addition to an annual income statement, some practices also have prepared a monthly and quarterly income statement. This is because they want to closely examine profits or losses during specific periods of operation.

The income statement will vary in complexity depending upon the business organization under examination. However, for purposes of

Anytown Physical Therapy
Income Statement

For the month ended November 30, 19XX

REVENUE

Services Performed		11,000
Allowances for Uncollectables (10%)		1,100
TOTAL REVENUE		$ 9,900

EXPENSES

Advertising	100	
Office Supplies	40	
Salaries	5,000	
Telephone	100	
Depreciation, Building	100	
Depreciation, Equipment	75	
Insurance	500	
Loan Repayment	1,000	
Taxes	1,000	
TOTAL EXPENSES		$ 7,915
NET INCOME		$ 1,985

Figure VI. This income statement shows that revenues during the month of November exceeded expenses and the practice earned a positive net income for the month. The advantage of using a monthly statement is it allows immediate assessment of down turns in practice income due to changes in operations.

simplicity, the income statement for a private practice can be best studied by including all practice operations into three categories; revenues, expenses, and net income.

Revenues are the receipts received by the practice during the period under examination. Revenue consists of money actually received from patients and additional amounts that are still due. For example, a patient treated today is recognized as revenue even though the patient may not make a payment for a month. The moment the practice provides health care to a patient, it can claim an increase in revenue.

Expenses are the costs of providing physical therapy services as an independent practitioner. Expenses can include any items used in the treatment of patients which cost the practice money. Examples include salaries, electricity, and insurance. In some situations, an expense such as insurance may not have to be paid for another sixty days. Nevertheless, it is still recorded as an expense during the period of time in which it was incurred.

Net income is the excess of practice revenue over expenses incurred during the period under examination. If revenue exceeds expenses, the practice has made a profit. If the opposite has occurred, then the practice has suffered a loss. In order to fully understand the income statement, it will be necessary to examine Figure VI. This is a simplified version of a monthly income statement from a private practice.

MAINTAINING FINANCIAL RECORDS

The process of properly maintaining financial records can be a very time-consuming activity. Records must be maintained in a manner which makes them easy to review by others, such as the Internal Revenue Service who may someday examine all accounts. Fortunately, there are a number of options available to assist the practitioner in maintaining proper financial records.

One option is to hire an accountant who comes in once a month and organizes the financial aspects of the practice. This can be quite expensive, and for many practitioners, it is the least desirable.

Another option is to hire a part-time retired person who comes in once a week to organize the books. Many of these individuals can provide expert financial guidance at extremely low hourly rates.

Finally, the owner of the practice can work closely with an employee to maintain proper records. This method has the advantage of allowing the practitioner to always remain aware of the financial situation of the practice. It does, however, have the disadvantage of taking a great deal of time away from patient treatment and practice management.

DETERMINING THE BREAK-EVEN POINT

There are many methods of financial analysis available for use in establishing a small business or private practice in physical therapy. One of the most simple to understand and utilize is the break-even model. The break-even model can be used by the practitioner as a guide to financial investment. The model will be of assistance in determining whether a practitioner's patient volume will be large enough to support the investment in the many types of rehabilitation equipment.

To understand the break-even model there must first be a definition of the break-even point. The break-even point is that point at which the practice revenue is equal to its cost of operation. By definition, the practice will lose money if the volume of patients needed is less than this amount and make a profit if the number of patients seen is greater than this amount.

In computing the break-even point for a private practice there are two types of costs that must be understood. These are fixed costs and variable costs.

A fixed cost is a practice expense which remains constant. Examples of fixed costs are rent, property taxes, and insurance. Each of these costs will remain constant or "fixed" for periods of about one year. These rates are fixed and do not change with increases or decreases of patient volume. If the practice has a good year or a bad year, the cost of rent and other fixed costs will not increase.

Variable costs are those expenses which change in relation to patient volume. When the practice treats only a few patients, these expenses will decrease. When the volume of patients increases, these expenses will also increase. For example; the more whirlpools performed by the practice, the higher the cost of the water bill, laundry bill, and electricity or gas bill to heat additional water. Reductions in the number of whirlpools provided will reduce each of these costs.

COMPUTING THE BREAK-EVEN POINT

In the following section, an illustration is provided for one of the simplest mathematical models for small business. The break-even model mathematically represents the relationship between the number of patient treatments, cost, and profit. It is simple to understand and relevent to many practice investment decisions.

For purposes of illustration, the patient treatment provided will be in its most elementary state. In this form, the practice will provide a specific treatment or service which costs the practice money. This treatment is labeled as a variable cost. A variable cost will "vary" because it will change in relation to changes in patient volume. Fixed costs are also incurred but do not change with the changes in patient volume. Profit will be thought of as total revenue less total cost.

When using mathematical models, it is often helpful to symbolically represent the items being modeled. In the example presented, the following symbols will be of importance.

P = Profit

R = Total Revenue

C = Total Cost

F = Fixed Cost

X = Number of patients receiving the treatment or service

S = The dollar amount the patient must pay per treatment or service

V = Cost to the practice per unit of treatment or service (Variable Cost)

Perhaps the best method to use in constructing a mathematical model for private practice is to first verbalize the many relationships. Once understood, the process can be transformed into a mathematical model.

"Total profit is obtained by the subtraction of total cost from total revenue."

Profit = Total Revenue – Total Cost

P = R – C

"Total revenue is obtained by multiplying the number of patients receiving the service by the dollar amount the patient must pay per treatment."

Total Revenue = number of patients times the dollar amount for service.

R = X · S

"Total cost is the sum of fixed and variable costs." The variable cost can be obtained by multiplying the number of patients receiving the service by the cost to the practice per unit of service.

Total Cost = Fixed cost + (Cost to the practice per unit of service times the number of patients receiving the service)

C = F + (V · X)

The relationships for profit, total cost and total revenue may be represented as follows:

$$P = R - C$$
$$P = SX - [F + VX]$$

The equation is now a simple mathematical model which can be utilized in practice operations. The model represents the various relationships between profit, dollar amount each patient pays per treatment, fixed cost, and the costs to the practice (variable costs) per patient. Its use can be illustrated in the following private practice example.

A practitioner purchased a continuous passive motion device for $3,750. It is estimated that each time the practice uses the machine for patient treatment it costs the practice $7.50. The $7.50 cost to the practice consists of employee time for setup, cleanup, and supplies used in treatment. The dollar amount charged to the patient for treatment is $25.00. Based on the information provided, the mathematical model can be used to answer several questions.

What will the profit be to the practice if four hundred patient treatments are provided?

$$P = SX - [F + VX]$$
$$P = 25(400) - [3750 + 7.50(400)]$$
$$P = 10,000 - [3750 + 3000] = \$3,250$$

How many patients must the practice treat in order to break even on the purchase of the machine? This implies the profit on the machine will be zero. The profit (P) must therefore be set equal to zero. Once set to zero the equation can then be solved for X, the number of patients who must receive treatment.

$$P = SX - [F + VX]$$
$$0 = 25X - [3750 + 7.50x]$$
$$0 = 17.5X - 3750$$
$$X = 214.28$$

In this example, simple algebra is used to analyze the investment problem. The practice would need to provide approximately two hundred and fifteen patient treatments to recover the $3,750 investment.

The break-even model has a number of advantages. It will allow the practitioner to analyze both the anticipated revenue from an investment and determine the number of patients a practice must see to obtain a return on investment. In some cases, after using the formula, you may find the cost of purchasing an expensive piece of equipment for patient treatment may take years to recover.

OBTAINING A LOAN FOR PRACTICE

Every practitioner needs money to begin and maintain ongoing operations in a private practice. Depending on the practice location, equipment needs, and staff size a practice will need anywhere from ten thousand dollars to twenty-five thousand dollars to begin operations. If you do not have sufficient funds to start a practice, you may decide to secure a loan from an individual or lending institution.

If you go to a lending institution, such as a bank, you will probably be considered for either an installment loan or a single payment loan. An installment loan is usually repaid on a monthly basis. The payment will be fixed at a predetermined interest rate. The single payment loan is repaid in its entirety on a specific date.

AMORTIZATION OF A LOAN

In many financial transactions with lending institutions a loan is considered discharged after making a series of payments. After making the last payment, the loan is said to have been amortized. Loans frequently amortized are those used for the purchase of home and automobiles.

Before deciding to obtain a loan investigate the cost of its repayment. This can be done by using a simple amortization formula. Although lending institutions vary on loan requirements and methods of repayment the formula will provide an estimate of how much it will cost the practitioner to borrow money at the prevailing interest rates.

THE AMORTIZATION FORMULA

In this section an illustration will be provided for one of the simplest mathematical models for loan repayment. As with other mathematical models it is often helpful to symbolically represent the items which will be under consideration.

R = the amount of the periodic payment

i = the interest rate

P = amount of the loan (principle)

N = total length of the loan

C = how often the loan is repaid (monthly, quarterly, or semi-annually, annually)

The amortization formula then becomes:

$$R = P \left[\frac{\frac{i}{C}}{1 - (1 + \frac{i}{C}) - N} \right]$$

For Example: If you were to obtain a five thousand dollar loan with a 9½ interest rate, how much would the monthly payment be if the entire loan was to be repaid in two years? The following will provide the solution.

P = 5000

N = (2 years)(12 months per year) = 24

i = .095

C = 12

Using the formula we have:

$$R = 5000 \left[\frac{\frac{.095}{12}}{1 - (1 + \frac{.095}{12}) - 24} \right]$$

$$R = 5000 \left[\frac{.00791667}{.17242196} \right]$$

R = 5000 [.04591449]

R = $229.57 per month

If, instead of a monthly payment the loan was to be repaid quarterly, how much would the quarterly payment be?

P = 5000

N = (2 years)(4 quarters per year) = 8

i = .095

C = 4

$$R = 5000 \left[\frac{\frac{.095}{4}}{1 - (1 + \frac{.095}{4} - 8} \right]$$

$$R = 5000 \left[\frac{.02375}{.17120} \right]$$

R = 5000 [.13872]

R $693.62 quarterly

If the loan is repaid at $693.62 on a quarterly basis, how much interest will be incurred? The total amount paid will be:

Eight quarters ($693.62 quarterly) = $5548.96

Of this amount, $548.96 is the interest.

The amortization formula has one major advantage. It allows the practitioner to determine how much of a loan can comfortably be afforded. Large monthly loan payments add to a practice's fixed costs. Do not try to buy everything the practice needs if it will cause an overload of debt. It is better to plan ahead than to buy simply because credit is easily available.

ADDITIONAL INFORMATION TO CONSIDER

If you decide the practice does need financial assistance, contact several lending institutions. In most lending institutions there is one individual who is responsible for making business loans to health care professionals. Prepare a brief financial statement prior to talking with this person. Specify the manner in which you intend to use the loan. Do not misrepresent your practice needs or how the money will be invested.

Depending upon the lending institution's assessment of your financial risk, you may be requested to provide collateral or have someone cosign the loan. In some cases, the equipment purchased with the loan can serve as collateral. In either situation, have a thorough understanding of how the loan may be used.

Before signing the loan agreement, investigate the prepayment or pay-off clauses. Some banks or lending institutions will assess a penalty for early retirement of a loan. If the loan agreement is unclear about the prepayment penalty, contact an attorney for clarification.

CHAPTER THREE

YOUR PRIVATE PRACTICE
INSURANCE NEEDS

THE SUBJECT of insurance should not be overlooked by the physical therapist who is embarking into the private practice setting. Even though the number of medical malpractice cases is decreasing, the size of jury awards is still increasing. Many states are trying to limit the damage amounts currently being awarded. Until legislative relief appears on the horizon, every physical therapist must have adequate insurance to protect his/her profession, business, and family against financial disaster.

It isn't financially possible to insure yourself, your business, and your family against every possible risk. Things are going to happen which you cannot foresee. You must, however, insure against risks that are foreseeable and could lead to financial devastation. This chapter discusses the basic insurance needs for a physical therapist in a private practice setting.

The insurance requirements for the private practitioner vary in complexity and ability to provide protection. There are three types of protection which are essential to all individuals who own a private practice. These are insurance programs which provide: (1) professional liability insurance (malpractice insurance) (2) practice and employee insurance, (3) protection for yourself and family.

PROFESSIONAL LIABILITY INSURANCE

Professional liability insurance protects you against legal actions alleging that you in some way wrongfully practiced physical therapy which resulted in a patient sustaining injury. These legal actions are an effort to compensate the injured patient for personal harm or financial loss.

In the medical profession, the cost to insure a practicing physical therapist has remained quite low. This is because the profession of physical therapy has sustained relatively few malpractice claims. Insurance companies set premium rates in accordance with the relative risk of the profession, and the number of outstanding malpractice cases against physical therapists.

Do not take this encouraging news to mean that, as a physical therapist, you do not need insurance. The decision to open a private practice without insurance to protect yourself is very risky. It may, at the very least, cost anywhere from twenty-five thousand to fifty thousand dollars to successfully defend a malpractice case. That sum must be paid by you unless you have obtained an insurance policy that provides for legal defense. Without professional liability insurance, your career could end in bankruptcy.

The amount of professional liability insurance you should carry may depend upon the area of the country in which you practice. Insurance companies recognize certain regions of the country as having greater risks due to a high number of malpractice claims. In these areas you may need to carry more insurance to adequately protect yourself. In general, physical therapy liability insurance which provides $100,000 per claim and $300,000 aggregate should provide sufficient protection. A policy with these provisions up to $100,000 per claim with no greater than three claims of malpractice per year. Of course, higher limits are available. You may prefer to have limits up to one million dollars.

Professional liability insurance has recently been changing. Many of the changes were a result of the losses insurance companies sustained due to large jury awards. Medical liability insurance now generally falls into two categories. These are called occurance and claims made policies.

Occurance Insurance Coverage

Occurance coverage is one of the oldest forms of liability insurance. An occurance policy protects the insured against claims arising from any treatment provided during the policy year. A claim under this form of coverage can be paid years after the policy was issued. Occurance policies carry what is known as the long tail effect.

The long tail effect provides coverage to the physical therapist long after retirement. The individual practitioner knows that once retired, the policy will provide coverage against any future claims.

The process of determining a premium for occurance coverage by the insurance company is difficult. It forces the company to plan for the long term. To set a price for an occurance policy, the company must be able to predict the social and economic changes in claims and recoveries which may occur in the future. Many companies have ceased offering these policies due to the increasing number of malpractice claims and rising jury awards.

Claims Made Policy

The claims made policy covers a physical therapist only against claims arising within the year the policy is in effect. Each year the practitioner must buy an endorsement of the policy which extends the period of coverage. The claims made policy is designed to avoid some of the difficulties posed by the long tail effect.

The claims made policy reduces the need for the company to plan for the long term. Insurance companies can protect themselves by requiring you to continue to purchase liability insurance for several years after you cease to practice.

PRACTICE AND EMPLOYEE INSURANCE

Public Liability Insurance

A physical therapist as owner of a private practice may be legally responsible for any accident or injury occuring on the premises which can be attributed to neglect. The responsibility for a patient's well being begins once the patient steps onto the land of the private practitioner. This includes the parking area and the steps used to gain entrance to the office.

Public liability insurance is designed to protect the practice from lawsuits as a result of injuries occuring on practice property. Policies in most cases can be written from $100,000 to $500,000. The advisability of purchasing this type of insurance depends most often on the type of patients who visit the facility. If your practice specializes in a patient group which requires the use of assistive devices (canes, walkers, crutches) there is likely to be a fall on the premises. With the prevalence of lawsuits today, it is recommended that this type of insurance coverage be purchased.

Auto Liability and Agency

As the owner of a private practice you have the legal distinction of being known as the principle. That designation means you have the authority to request employees or agents to act on your behalf. The principle/agent relationship is one area often overlooked in liability insurance.

In a private practice, quite often employees perform services which require the use of an automobile. These services may simply involve driving to a local store to obtain supplies for the office. If the employee is involved in an auto accident while performing a service for the practice and found to be negligent, a recovery for damages could be made against the employee and the owner of the car or practice.

There are four types of auto liability insurance which must be investigated by the practitioner. They are: (1) property damage liability insurance, (2) bodily injury liability insurance, (3) medical payments insurance, (4) collision insurance.

Property damage insurance provides protection against damage to another individual's property as a result of an auto accident. Bodily injury liability insurance provides coverage to anyone who suffers personal injury because of the accident. Medical payments insurance covers the medical needs of those individuals inside the vehicle.

Collision insurance helps to pay the cost of repairing the automobile after the accident. There are two types of coverage; full and deductible. Under full or complete coverage all costs to repair a vehicle are paid by the insurance company. The deductible coverage pays the full cost of repairs after the deductible has been met. Most practitioners have either a one-hundred or five-hundred dollar deductible. Full coverage has the highest premium costs, therefore the higher the deductible, the lower the cost of the premium.

Practice Fire Insurance

Office fires are less common today than in years past. With the advent of the smoke detector, sprinkler systems, security systems, and improvements in electrical systems the likelihood of a fire and smoke damage is decreasing. Even with the scientific advancements, the private practitioner should still carry fire insurance. Practice fire insurance should cover not only the value of the building but also the value of the equipment.

Depending on the insurance company, individual policies may require you to carry insurance limits equal to eighty, ninety, or even one hundred percent of the total value of the structure. If there is a fire, you will be required to pay the difference between the actual coverage and the percentage you chose not to carry. It is important for the beginning practitioner to have all items one hundred percent covered. Very few practitioners could afford to start over if the building and its contents were completely destroyed.

Perform a yearly inventory of all items (equipment and furnishings) contained in the office. Many insurance companies suggest you photograph all aspects of the inside and outside of the office. Frequently, those items which do not show up on an inventory list can be spotted in a photograph. Keep both the inventory and photographs in a safe place. Do not store them in the office.

Fire insurance is also available to cover areas other than the building and equipment. Patient medical records and accounts receivable can easily be destroyed in a fire. Insurance can be purchased to cover both of these items or the practitioner can invest in a fireproof safe for their protection.

Further protection can be afforded by purchasing business interruption insurance. A private practice may suffer financially if forced to move to a temporary office without the use of valuable equipment. Business interruption insurance will pay the practitioner for lost income because of damage to the office or equipment.

Employee Theft Insurance

As the practice grows and begins to do financially well, there is potential for large sums of money to exchange hands between office personnel and the patients seen for treatment. Although you may believe you have done an excellent job of selecting practice personnel, sometimes the temptation to take money belonging to the practice can be overwhelming.

One way of protecting a practice from this possibility is to use fidelity bonds. Fidelity bonds can be written to cover a specific person, position, or group. If there is financial loss due to employee embezzlement, the insurance company will pay up to the amount specified in the policy.

Worker's Compensation Insurance

All states, including the federal government, have adopted workers compensation laws. Under these laws, employees who are injured on the job are entitled to fair compensation. Each state has a law which defines the extent to which an employer is financially responsible for the death, disability, or medical expenses of an employee who suffers an occupational injury or illness.

The benefits provided under workers' compensation are two types: medical and income. Some states require complete medical payments while others place a limit on medical benefits.

Under workers compensation, provisions have been made for the rehabilitation training programs to allow individuals who cannot return to their former jobs to be trained for new occupations. Income compensation amounts may vary, but often pay as much as two-thirds of the employee's average salary up to a maximum limit. To lower the administrative costs of small injuries and prevent an employee from fabricating an injury to obtain a holiday, many insurance companies pay nothing to compensate wage loss from two to seven days following the injury.

Workers compensation laws vary from state to state. The relevance of the law to your practice frequently depends upon the number of employees. Since most practitioners must have this insurance, consult your insurance agent for information regarding your practice situation.

Insurance to Cover Overhead Expenses

During short periods of practitioner disability, the employees can still carry on the activities of billing and collecting on patient accounts. Overhead expenses include such items as employee salaries and office rent which must be paid to keep the office functioning.

The benefits paid on office overhead insurance are based on established office expenses. They are not based on practice income, and will only be continued until such time as you can resume practice.

PROTECTION FOR YOURSELF AND FAMILY

Disability Insurance for the Owner

The beginning private practitioner is the individual who organizes, manages, and directs the flow of income to the practice. Any injury which prevents a practitioner from evaluating and treating patients for a long period of time could jeopardize his/her personal financial stability. Every individual practitioner should consider purchasing disability insurance. A severe injury which required the practitioner to be away from the business for a long period of time could result in lost personal earnings not recoverable, in some cases, for months or years.

Disability insurance is designed to replace income lost as a result of an extended injury or illness. Most policies are written to replace part, but not all, of your income. Policies are generally one of three types. They can be cancellable, for a guaranteed period, or guaranteed renewable.

Cancellable policies are generally the least desirable. They can be cancelled by the insurance company at any time during which a premium has been paid and accepted. The guaranteed period disability insurance is more favorable since it is noncancellable during the period in which the premium was paid and accepted. The guaranteed renewable is noncalcellable as long as each premium is paid by the practitioner. It can be renewed each year up to a maximum age.

Many factors influence the cost of disability insurance. The cost is most often influenced by the length of time benefits are to be paid out, and the waiting period between the onset of the disability and the beginning of disability payment. Policies can be written for almost any waiting period. The choice of a waiting period (thirty, sixty, ninety, or three-hundred and sixty days) must be determined after assessing how long you, the individual practitioner, could survive with little or no income. If you are an individual practitioner, disability benefits are nontaxable. In group practices, disability payments may be taxable if premiums were paid as part of the general business expenses.

Should Life Insurance Be Included?

Life insurance is one of the oldest forms of insurances available. The purpose of life insurance is to pay benefits to family members, fellow practice associates, or creditors in the event of your death. Life insurance can be very helpful to a small partnership practice that would like to continue operation in the event one partner dies. If one partner dies, and the practice is named beneficiary, the fellow associates could use the proceeds to purchase the individual's interest in the practice and continue operation. Although there are many different policies available to the practitioner, the two most common are term life insurance and ordinary or whole life insurance.

Term life insurance provides coverage only for a specified number of years. The premium cost for this insurance is usually quite low. In most cases it will not provide for loan values or a cash surrender value. The primary disadvantage to term insurance is that the cost of the policy will rise with age. Many insurance companies do, however, offer a plan to convert to a more permanent insurance within a certain period of time.

WHOLE LIFE INSURANCE ILLUSTRATION

MALE PREFERRED AGE 31

FACE AMOUNT: $100000

ANNUAL PREMIUM: $621.00

				GUARANTEED INTEREST 5.5			CURRENT INTEREST 9.3%		
YEAR	AGE	ANNUAL PAYMENT	TOTAL PAYMENTS	SURR VAL**	CASH VALUE	DEATH BENEFIT	SURR VAL**	CASH VALUE	DEATH BENEFIT
1	31	621	621	0	406	100000	0	437	100000
2	32	621	1242	0	836	100000	0	915	100000
3	33	621	1863	0	1290	100000	38	1438	100000
4	34	546	2409	284	1684	100000	523	1923	100000
5	35	546	2954	688	2088	100000	1041	2441	100000
6	36	546	3500	1395	2515	100000	1888	3008	100000
7	37	546	4046	2115	2955	100000	2777	3617	100000
8	38	546	4592	2848	3408	100000	3726	4286	100000
9	39	546	5137	3594	3874	100000	4855	5135	100000
10	40	546	5683	4344	4344	100000	6040	6040	100000
11	41	0	5683	4299	4299	100000	6476	6476	100000
12	42	0	5683	4227	4227	100000	6944	6944	100000
13	43	0	5683	4139	4139	100000	7447	7447	100000
14	44	0	5683	4022	4022	100000	7986	7986	100000
15	45	0	5683	3875	3875	100000	8565	8565	100000
16	46	0	5683	3695	3695	100000	9178	9178	100000
17	47	0	5683	3470	3470	100000	9828	9828	100000
18	48	0	5683	3207	3207	100000	10519	10519	100000
19	49	0	5683	2893	2893	100000	11250	11250	100000
20	50	0	5683	2524	2524	100000	12024	12024	100000
21	51	0	5683	2085	2085	100000	12884	12884	100000
22	52	0	5683	1571	1571	100000	13798	13798	100000
23	53	0	5683	964	964	100000	14769	14769	100000
24	54	0	5683	247	247	100000	15799	15799	100000
25	55	0	5683	0	0	0	16890	16890	100000
26	56	0	5683	0	0	0	18045	18045	100000
27	57	0	5683	0	0	0	19268	19268	100000
28	58	0	5683	0	0	0	20566	20566	100000
29	59	0	5683	0	0	0	21942	21942	100000
30	60	0	5683	0	0	0	23408	23408	100000
31	61	0	5683	0	0	0	24970	24970	100000
32	62	0	5683	0	0	0	26635	26635	100000
33	63	0	5683	0	0	0	28409	28409	100000
34	64	0	5683	0	0	0	30301	30301	100000
35	65	0	5683	0	0	0	32323	32323	100000
36	66	0	5683	0	0	0	34486	34486	100000
37	67	0	5683	0	0	0	36810	36810	100000
38	68	0	5683	0	0	0	39319	39319	100000
39	69	0	5683	0	0	0	42045	42045	100000
40	70	0	5683	0	0	0	45023	45023	100000
41	71	0	5683	0	0	0	48269	48269	100000
42	72	0	5683	0	0	0	51822	51822	100000
43	73	0	5683	0	0	0	55726	55726	100000
44	74	0	5683	0	0	0	60038	60038	100000
45	75	0	5683	0	0	0	64837	64837	100000
46	76	0	5683	0	0	0	70212	70212	100000
47	77	0	5683	0	0	0	76273	76273	100000
48	78	0	5683	0	0	0	83141	83141	100000
49	79	0	5683	0	0	0	90990	90990	100000
50	80	0	5683	0	0	0	100006	100006	100000

** REPRESENTS CASH VALUE LESS SURRENDER CHARGES

Figure VII. This is a policy for a thirty-one-year-old male in good health. Under this policy, annual payments are made for ten years after which the policy is considered paid up. The minimum interest paid under this policy is 5.5%. The money is, however, invested by the company at a 9.3% current market rate.

Ordinary life insurance, sometimes called whole life insurance, offers the practitioner a combination of protection and savings. Ordinary life insurance is available in two forms. You can purchase life insurance that is considered fully paid after a specified number of annual premiums have been made or until you reach a certain age.

If the practice members are young, ordinary life insurance may be the most economical. Although the premiums may be higher than under term insurance, the policy will build up what is called cash surrender value. Cash surrender value is money which is payable to the policyholder upon cancellation of the policy. Many of these policies will allow you to borrow against the cash surrender value at a low rate of interest.

Employee Group Insurance Plans

In order for the practitioner to attract potential employees to the facility, it is often necessary to offer a large number of benefits. One of the benefits frequently offered in private practice is group insurance. Group insurance policies are usually one-year, renewable term policies. The practitioner commonly pays at least a portion of the premium with the employee paying the remainder.

Group insurance can offer life, health, dental, disability, and retirement programs. The insuring company frequently requires no physical examination since it makes no selection of the individuals who will be insured. Premiums are based solely on the characteristics of the group as a whole. Many companies do, however, require a minimum number of employees. This is to guard against risk and lower administrative costs.

Health Insurance

Almost all group insurance plans chosen for the private practice setting include some form of health insurance. This type of insurance is important for two reasons. First, as mentioned, group insurance can be used to attract prospective employees to a facility. It helps the individual practitioner to remain competitive. Second, insurance as a group is generally much less expensive than individual insurance plans. Group plans allow the practitioner to obtain coverage for themselves and family as well as providing individual employees with fringe benefits.

There are a number of health plans available. The most common group insurance plan is the comprehensive medical insurance. The comprehensive policy provides coverage to the primary areas of medical care needed in the event of an accident or illness. Comprehensive plans generally include:

1. Hospital Insurance. Most plans have a maximum allowable room charge per day and a specified number of days of hospitalization.

2. Surgical Expense Insurance. This insurance covers all necessary surgery as a result of an injury or illness. Many plans require second opinions before surgery and do not provide for plastic surgery unrelated to the injury or illness.

3. Physician Insurance. This insurance can be called basic insurance. It combines both hospital and surgical insurance. Physician insurance provides for nonsurgical care including physician office visits.

4. Major Medical Insurance. Major medical insurance plans are designed to cover an array of physician, hospital, laboratory, and nursing services beyond the limits of the basic plan. Their primary purpose is to pay medical expenses even if the person is not hospitalized. In most cases, deductibles must be met before benefits are paid by the insurance company. Deductibles can range from one-hundred to one-thousand dollars. Most insurance companies will pay 80 percent of the cost, beyond the deductible, with the employee paying the remaining 20 percent.

Mortgage Insurance

As your practice and family grows, you will begin to acquire additional personal assets. One of the assets purchased may include a home. Prices for new homes are still rising with many monthly mortgage payments approximating one-thousand to fifteen-hundred dollars.

In the event of your unexpected death, your family could have great difficulty in meeting a large monthly payment. Many insurance companies now offer homeowner mortgage insurance. Upon death, the balance of the mortgage would be paid by the insurance company. The premium costs for this insurance will vary depending on the size of the outstanding mortgage and the age of the homeowner.

Determining What Is Best for You

Many factors must be considered when purchasing insurance. Do not attempt to make all the decisions without professional guidance. Consult several insurance agents who can offer recommendations for personal and practice insurance. Compare prices and policies.

When considering the acceptance of a staff position in a private practice, ask for a full explanation of the insurance benefit programs. In some practice situations, there may be a limited benefit period or probationary period when no insurance will be provided. If this is the case, you may need to acquire insurance elsewhere until such time as you are adequately covered by the practice.

CHAPTER FOUR

PLACING A VALUE
ON A PHYSICAL THERAPY PRACTICE

ARRIVING at an appropriate value for a physical therapy practice is a complex process. Many tangible and intangible factors must be examined to properly gauge a practice value. As more individual practices are established, there will be increasing opportunities to purchase or become a partner in an established practice.

Evaluating the financial performance of any business is not an easy process. Many attempts have been made to develop specific formulas to assist in determining productivity in a practice as well as overall practice value. None of these formulas, nor the ones to be presented, are inclusive. They can only serve as guides to areas of a private practice which must be carefully examined prior to purchase.

The formulas and areas examined in this chapter are intended to acquaint the reader with methods to evaluate private practice financial performance. Do not use these as the sole means of evaluating a practice prior to purchase. For an investment of this type you will need to seek advice from a tax attorney, certified public accountant, or professional management consultant.

PURCHASING AN ONGOING PRACTICE

One of the easiest ways of getting into private practice is to purchase an ongoing practice. A great number of problems associated with opening a new practice can be avoided by using this method. Problems with establishing a patient load, hiring and training employees, and developing a cash flow can all be greatly simplified.

The purchase of practice is, however, not a simple process. A private practice is a collection of many assets, each of which must be valued separately. The prospective practitioner must be willing to spend a considerable amount of time negotiating the purchase price of each asset. Once individual assets are valued, they can be summed to the total purchase price of the practice.

ADVANTAGES OF PURCHASING AN ONGOING PRACTICE

There are a number of advantages to purchasing an ongoing practice. Four of the most important are:

1. Since the practice is established, there is less risk of financial failure.
2. The planning normally required to start a new practice is greatly reduced.
3. The practice may be for sale at a very reasonable cost.
4. The established practice does not have to develop a practice market.

Each of these four advantages is discussed in detail below.

Lower Rate of Financial Failure

There are two potential problems that face the physical therapist who opens a new practice. First, there is the risk that the practice will be unable to meet rent, salary, and other practice costs. Second, there is the risk that patients will not become aware or choose to utilize your health care services. If either of these situations occurs, the practice could end in financial failure.

The purchase of an existing practice helps to reduce the chances of either event. An established practice generally has a proven record of attracting patients, effectively controlling costs, and making a profit.

The purchase of an existing practice also eliminates the sometimes very difficult decision of where to locate. This question has already been successfully determined by the existing owner. The owner has probably spent a great deal of personal time and money advertising and acquainting the community with services offered by the practice. The practice is, therefore, already well known.

Reduction of Planning

The established practitioner has already brought together the efficient combinations of personnel and equipment to make the practice a success. Getting the "right group" of employees together and making a profit can be a difficult process.

The new practitioner must spend considerable time planning and communicating the practice direction to new employees. When purchasing an established practice, it is generally expected that the nucleus of the practice staff will remain. As long as the new owner treats the staff fairly, less time and effort will be required to develop practice personnel and communicate objectives and goals.

Reasonable Cost

Many variables can influence why the owner of the practice wants to sell. For example, the owner may be forced to sell the practice due to either personal or health reasons. It is also possible that the owner has located another practice opportunity which he/she would rather pursue. In either instance, the present owner may be willing to sell at a lower price simply to get out from under the present practice responsibilities.

There are very few occasions when a practice will be priced below market value. The physical therapist selling the practice has a proven record of skillful business and professional practices. It is, however, to your advantage to be well versed in knowing what to look for in practice opportunities.

Practice Market

One of the most important areas that must be examined prior to opening a new practice is the practice market. Determining a practice market means to identify the specific group of patients you would like to attract to the office. Purchasing an established practice lessens this burden. The present owner has already worked very hard at attracting both a first time and a repeat volume of patients.

The purchase of an established practice will also provide the opportunity to expand into other areas of practice interest. When evaluating a practice for possible purchase, the strengths and weakness of the practice should become evident. After purchase, the practice can be further enhanced by developing marketing strategies to correct for any weaknesses in the provision of health care.

For example, the prospective practice may be a leader in providing health care to orthopaedic patients. Through further community analysis, it may become evident that the needs of neurological patients are not being satisfied. With the orthopaedic practice well established, the practitioner could direct attention towards the neurological patient market.

QUESTIONS WHICH MUST BE ASKED

In the process of evaluating and deciding whether or not to purchase a practice the prospective owner must ask and receive answers to several important questions. The following four questions provide a guide to analysis.

Why Is the Practice for Sale?

There must first be an attempt to determine why the owner is selling the practice. In many situations, there may be a significant difference between the answer given and the real reason. Answers such as, "I think it may be time to retire" can be very evasive. When personal answers are vague, the prospective owner must look at business-related information.

Ask where the owner intends to relocate after the practice is sold. It is possible, for example, for an established practitioner to move across town and set up a new practice next to another hospital. This could be disastrous if the owner's established patients also moved with the practice.

Situations such as these can be avoided by having the owner agree to enter into a contract not to compete. Noncompetition contracts of this type should clearly spell out the number of years and distance away that any new practice may be established.

Also inquire about potential changes at the present location. Is the current lease about to expire? Does the building have major structural or electrical problems? Did the owner recently receive information indicating the present lease would not be renewed? Who is responsible for the cost of any improvements made to the building?

What Is the Condition of the Medical Equipment?

Carefully examine all equipment which is to be sold with the practice. Both furniture and equipment may represent a large portion of the practice value. The value of these items depends upon how old they are, how soon they will have to be replaced, and their future maintenance requirements. Ask to see purchase receipts and service records on all equipment.

Equipment or furniture which is rented or leased by the seller cannot be included as a practice asset. However, if the lease is assumable it may be in the best interest of the buyer to negotiate a price for the assumption opportunity. Make sure the company leasing the equipment approves the transaction in writing.

Will the Employees Remain?

The physical therapist who established the practice is probably the most important asset. This individual brought together the necessary financial and nonfinancial resources to make the practice a success. There are, however, key employees who also contributed to the success of the practice. Unfortunately, some of these employees may have plans to leave once the practice is sold.

If it is evident that a large portion of key personnel are leaving the practice, there must be a reduction from the purchase price. The reduction is to allow for the recruitment and training of new personnel. In some practice situations it may take six months to one year to replace a physical therapist or physical therapy assistant. A loss of an employee for that length of time can be costly to a new practitioner.

What Type of Competition Is There?

The health care industry is very competitive. Regardless of the quality of medical care provided, there is always a limit to the number of people who will need it and how much they will spend. The more private practices located in the same region, the stronger the competition to provide health care services. The larger the number of practitioners, the greater the costs of advertising to reach the market. Increasing competition ultimately means lower practice profits.

Knowing the competition means thoroughly understanding the environment of the medical community. It is essential that the prospective owner determine the direction of community growth. Find out where the patients go to receive physical therapy and who refers them there. A good number of patients seek physical therapy at the recommendation of their doctor. These same patients may also be instructed to receive therapy at specific locations. The seller of the practice may know the direction of community growth and want to sell before profits begin to drop.

WHAT IS THE FINANCIAL OUTLOOK FOR THE PRACTICE?

When purchasing a private practice it is important to acquire the professional services of either a certified public accountant (C.P.A.) or a tax attorney. These individuals are skilled at assessing the financial performance of a business. They will examine a number of areas of interest and then offer their opinion as to the financial stability of the practice.

Professionals know that simply examining the records and books is not enough to determine the financial performance and stability of a practice. The attorney or C.P.A. should closely examine the bank deposits for the last several years. If the practice has only been in possession of the current owner for a short period of time, ask to see the financial records of the previous owner. It is also within reason to request a copy of the owner's tax returns. After all, it is your money that will be invested. You need to know as much information about the practice as can be obtained.

Closely examine the practice's profit trend. If the practice is growing, profits should reflect it. It could be quite possible that the practice is not growing despite everything the seller has done to increase it. Determine if more is spent on advertising each year, but profits remain unchanged. The practitioner may be selling the practice simply because it is only making a small annual profit.

Through careful examination, it is possible to determine how well a practice is doing. If the financial performance has been good, and it appears to be solid for the future, you then need to begin assessing the price.

HOW MUCH SHOULD I PAY?

The price to be paid for the practice should reflect a fair profit for the seller and a reasonable cost for the buyer. Determining the final price can be a difficult process, especially since there are no absolute formulas to use in analysis. There are, however, some specific areas which warrant attention. The nine most important are:

1. Previous earnings
2. Accounts receivable
3. Goodwill
4. Building improvements
5. Supplies and inventory
6. Leases
7. Equipment
8. Prepaid expenses
9. Real estate

Previous Earnings

Previous earnings are important because they reflect one of the primary reasons to establish a private practice, that is, to make money. Many economic and noneconomic factors can influence the profit picture of a practice. It should, however, be making a profit in order to be under serious consideration.

Accounts Receivable

Accounts receivable is an asset to the practice representing a dollar amount owed by the patients for medical services. The value of accounts receivable is influenced by many factors. They are, however, very seldom if ever equal to their face value.

The older the patient's account, the less value it has. It decreases in value with age because there is less likelihood that it will ever be paid. Turning past due accounts over to a collection agency further diminishes their value because most agencies will only pay the practice half of what they collect.

Examine how quickly the practitioner has made collections in the past. If collection results have not been good, it is unlikely that your attempts to collect on old accounts will demonstrate any improvement.

Consider the following possibilities when purchasing accounts receivable:

1. Purchase all accounts receivable after they have been discounted for age.
2. Allow the seller to retain accounts receivable and collect them.
3. The buyer can agree to attempt the collection of accounts receivable for a dollar percentage of what is collected.

Goodwill

The prospective practitioner must also examine the intangible asset of goodwill. Goodwill is the value the seller places on the practice above what the accounting statements indicate. It involves the assumption that patients will continue to seek medical services of the practice once it has been sold.

Goodwill can be influenced by many factors. Some of the most important to consider are:

1. How long it would take to set up a similar practice.
2. The financial risk of opening a new practice.

3. The amount of income that can be made purchasing an existing practice rather than starting a new one.
4. The price of the goodwill under consideration as compared to the price of goodwill of other similar practices.
5. The value placed on the seller agreeing not to set up a competing practice.
6. The assistance the seller will provide once you take control of the practice.

The willingness of the seller to assist in the retention of employees is also a key factor. The seller may agree to stay on as a consultant until you become comfortable with practice operations. It is important to remember, however, that the buyer cannot see goodwill, but must make every attempt to assess it and assign an appropriate value.

Building Improvements

Some small value can be added for building improvements. It is important, however, to examine the lease. In some leases it may specify that improvements become property of the building owner.

Supplies and Inventory

If supplies and inventory are usable, buy them at the price the owner originally paid. If they are slow moving, adjust the price downward. If prices have risen, adjust the price to reflect the change.

Leases

If a lease is long term and favorable, it can be an asset to the selling price. If there is a provision to sublease and conditions are favorable both the seller and buyer may benefit.

Equipment

Take the original purchase price less the amount of accumulated depreciation. Depreciation can be determined through an examination of previous tax returns.

Prepaid Expenses

These include fire and liability insurance paid on an annual basis. They can be purchased at cost.

Real Estate

If the seller of the practice owns the land and building where the practice is located, it may also be for sale. On the other hand, the seller may wish to retain the building and property and establish a rental agreement. The rental agreement should be separate from the purchase of the practice.

Valuating a Practice

There are a number of formulas which could be used to assess the value of a private practice. In most cases, your attorney or CPA will use a formula which they have found acceptable for medical practice valuation. The following describes one uncomplicated and straightforward method to use for the financial analysis of a private practice.

VALUATING A PRACTICE

1. ASSETS		
Furniture		$ 10,000
Medical Equipment		120,000
Office Supplies		3,000
Other		1,000
		$134,000
2. Debts		
Outstanding Loan		$ 40,000
3. VALUE OF BUSINESS		$ 94,000
4. OWNER'S SALARY	$ 35,000	
5. PROJECTED PROFIT	40,000	
6. EXTRA EARNINGS	$ 5,000	
7. GOODWILL		$ 48,000
8. TOTAL PRICE		$142,000

9. $48,000 ÷ $5,000 = 9.6 YEARS

Figure VIII.

Step One: Determine the value of all practice assets. If any furniture or medical equipment is leased, it should not be included as an asset. The value of all assets should reflect depreciation. Depreciation is an estimate of the amount of the original cost that has been used as a result of wear or obsolescence. The total value of all assets after depreciation is $134,000.

Step Two: Calculate all the debts owed by the practice. These debts will be assumed by the new practice owner. Debts consist of one loan of $40,000.

Step Three: Subtract step two from step one. This gives a rough estimate of the value of the business. In this case the figure is $94,000.

Step Four: Determine the salary you would make as owner. This figure should reflect what you could make as a department director at another facility.

Step Five: Calculate the projected profit before taxes and before subtracting the owner's salary.

Step Six: Subtract the owner's salary (step four) from the projected profit (step five). This figure represents the extra money the physical therapist will earn from being in private practice. In this instance, it is $5,000.

Step Seven: Assess the reasonableness of the seller's value for goodwill. In this practice, the value has been set at $48,000. Is this a good value? Further calculation is needed.

Step Eight: Total price. Determined by adding step three and step seven. The total is $142,000.

Step Nine: Determine if the value of goodwill is too high by dividing the value of goodwill ($48,000) by the projected extra annual earnings ($5,000). It has been determined that it will take over nine and one half years to obtain a return on investment. This figure would be considered too high. In a well established practice, five years is considered a reasonable period to wait to obtain a return on investment. If the practice is somewhat younger, then one to three years may be appropriate. In this situation, the value of goodwill may be as much as $23,000 too high. This practice should be valued more closely to $119,000 to be under serious consideration.

One advantage of this formula is that it is of benefit in determining the appropriate asking price for goodwill. In the practice situation presented, the owner's salary was less than the projected profit before subtracting the owner's salary. This can be verified by comparing steps four and five. The latter is $5,000 larger. If the latter was not larger, then little if any value should be assigned to the intangible asset of goodwill. This is because the buyer can earn more from working elsewhere than could be earned from owning a private practice.

When presented with this situation, the buyer must proceed with caution. It is unlikely the seller will allow the practice to be purchased for only the value of the assets minus the liabilities. Some middle ground must be negotiated. It will be imperative for the buyer to determine what changes must be made to make the practice profitable before settling on an appropriate price for goodwill.

PLACING A VALUE ON INDIVIDUAL PRODUCTIVITY IN A GROUP PRACTICE

Measuring individual member productivity in a group practice and designing a fair compensation program can be a difficult task. Each group member wants assurance that they are being paid fairly for the work they are doing. No member of the group wants to profit at the expense of another.

There are a number of ideas on how to develop the perfect compensation formula. This formula does not represent the ideal. It does, however, provide a means to evaluate possible productivity problems between individual members in a group practice.

In some private practices, income is divided equally. This can present the worst of all situations. No two physical therapist's are equally productive. It will soon become apparent to the members of a group that one individual works somewhat slower than everyone else, and as a result does not bring in as much revenue to the practice.

Other practices distribute income based upon the percentage of total revenue generated by each practice member. This is a more equitable method, but it fails to allocate expenses appropriately. In many practice situations the physical therapist who sees the greatest number of patients also has the highest usage of office supplies, linen, employee assistance, and postage.

The basis for examining productivity in a practice need not be difficult. In the example, fixed costs are shared equally. These expenses include office rent and insurance. Fixed costs remain the same. They do not change with changes in patient volume. Variable expenses fluctuate in direct relationship to the productivity of the therapist. The more patients a therapist sees, the greater the cost of supplies, postage, and so on. Variable expenses can be tied directly to the percentage of individual patient billings. The method presented, although simplified, does present a more equitable compensation between group members.

INCOME FOR YEAR 19XX

	Total	Therapist "A"	Therapist "B"
Net Charges	$175,000	$125,000	$50,000
% of Total Charges	100%	71.4%	28.6%
Fixed Costs	$ 64,000	$ 32,000	$32,000
Variable Costs	$ 27,000	$ 19,278	$ 7,722
TOTAL COSTS	$ 91,000	$ 51,278	$39,722
Overhead Ratio	52%	41%	79.4%
Therapist Salary	$ 80,000	$ 40,000	$40,000
NET INCOME (LOSS)	$ 4,000	$ 33,722	($29,722)

Figure IX. Clearly there is a problem in this practice. Therapist "A" is supporting almost the entire practice. If Therapist "B" were in an individual practice, there would soon be bankruptcy proceedings. In this simplified case, Therapist "B" had been out of work due to a prolonged illness. This is, however, a good example of how a group practice could be abused if not monitored.

CHAPTER FIVE

THE LEGAL ASPECTS
OF PRIVATE PRACTICE

THE DAILY operation of an out patient facility requires a specialized knowledge of business law. As a private practitioner, you are not only responsible for the daily treatment of patients, but also for the operation of a business which must conform to the laws of the state.

As your practice grows and becomes established in a community, the legal profession may seek out your specialized opinion concerning the medical condition of a patient that you are currently treating or treated at one time. It is at your advantage to know how to react to the countless demands which can be made of your time by individuals outside of the practice.

This chapter examines the process of how you, as an individual business person, can become involved in the legal process. It discusses the principles of proper record handling, providing testimony, and discharging a patient from medical services. It is not a complete legal guide, but instead, an overview of the principles to follow until such time as you can seek the advice of legal council.

THE IMPORTANCE OF MEDICAL RECORDS

The importance of medical records which contain all relevant information and are accurate cannot be overemphasized. The great majority of malpractice cases that end in favor of the defendant do so because the defendant had witnesses and records that attest to the acceptable professional standard of performance in health care.

In many states it can take as long as five years to reach a court with a malpractice claim. It is therefore important that all records maintained in your office contain sufficient information which will allow you to fully recall the details of the treatment and the response of the patient to the treatment provided. It is very important that records contain a documentation of treatment in chronological sequence. Any alteration of a medical record, no matter how insignificant it may be, could be used against you in a court of law. It is frequently implied that you did something wrong. Proper record keeping is essential to building a good defense in a malpractice issue.

Some physical therapists have begun photographing a patient prior to treatment. This is done not only to document improvement but also in case an important issue should arise years later. A photograph serves to assist the therapist's memory of a prior treatment.

It is generally best to follow a consistant pattern in all record keeping. You should at least include the following information on all patients seen in the practice.

1. The history of the accident/injury/illness. Also include, using as much of the patient's own words as possible, a complete description of the medical problem.
2. A report of your physical examination of the patient.
3. Your impression of the patient's present ailment.
4. The treatment you recommend or performed.

If any of your findings differ significantly from the attending physician's diagnosis, contact him/her at once. Do not offer any treatment until you have thoroughly discussed the case with the physician. It is important to also document the conversation you had with the physician and ask for a revised referral form.

THE FILING SYSTEM FOR MEDICAL RECORDS

A daily procedure for record keeping should be established early in practice. It is generally best to keep the notes you make on a patient separate from their financial records. Although it may appear to be a much more convenient system, it frequently becomes very troublesome when you must compete with the receptionist for a chart while she is trying to bill the patient. It is also unwise to expose confidential patient notes to individuals, such as collection agencies, who someday may examine the accounts.

All records should be filed where they are easily accessible. The information about a patient should be organized in an individual folder clearly marked with the patient's name. Investigate the cost of obtaining fireproof filing cabinets for all records. The cost of replacing fire or smoke damaged records can be very expensive.

When looking for medical record filing cabinets, consider what filing space your practice will need as it grows. Many offices have installed open shelf cabinets because they take up less space than the conventional drawer file. If you decide to use cabinet files, keep in mind that they can serve as room dividers. Desks can be placed between files to allow for more individual privacy.

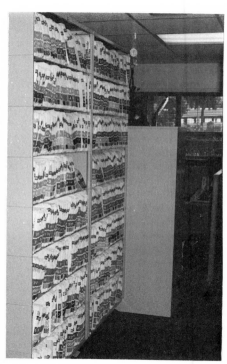
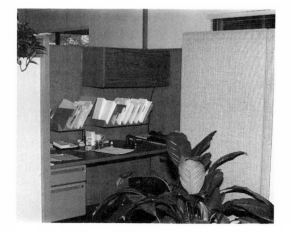

Figure X. Open shelf cabinets can hold hundreds of patient records and make it much easier to locate a patient record rather than the usage of a conventional filing system. The proper use of filing cabinets can allow the creation of an office within an office.

Some private practitioners have begun using the more modern color coded charting system. This system may also be incorporated with the standard numerical system. In either system the patient's record should be designed to be filed or pulled quickly and easily by all staff members.

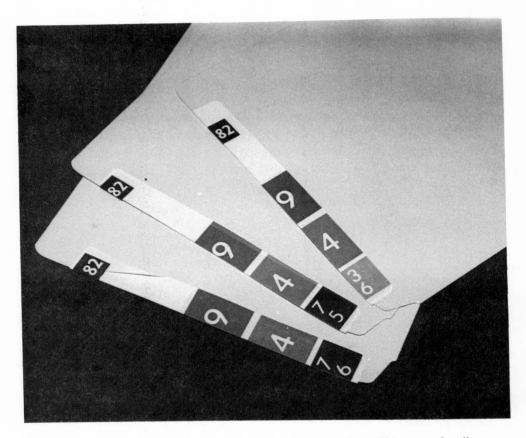

Figure XI. Patient records can be color coded and numerical. This type of coding can also indicate the year the record was created to enable files that are no longer active to be easily located and removed.

As the practice grows you may wish to thin your files by eliminating those charts which contain the records of patients no longer treated by the practice. In most states, medical records must be kept available for a period of five years after the last visit. If you desire to keep a copy of the records beyond that period of time, you may wish to consider microfilming them. This is generally a very expensive process but has the advantage of freeing up a large percentage of your filing cabinet space.

More and more private practitioners are dictating their medical findings and having them transcribed into the record rather than using the time consuming process of hand writing them. Depending on how busy your practice becomes, this can be a cost effective service. The average private practitioner may spend well over one hour per day hand writing notes or letters. This is time during which patient treatments cannot be performed.

RELEASE OF MEDICAL RECORDS

Medical records contain confidential information regarding treatment provided to a patient. They belong to the physical therapist and the facility where treatment was provided. They do not belong to the patient. Information contained in the patient record should be carefully protected from individuals not involved in patient care. Records should only be transferred from the office after receiving written authorization from the patient. You should always retain the original copy of the authorization form as well as the original medical records. All patient information should be kept in the patient's permanent file.

You may charge a small fee for the administrative costs of copying the records. Fees of up to three dollars are acceptable depending upon the length of time involved and the volume of the records to be copied. Postage should be the patient's responsibility.

RECORDS RELEASE

Date _____

To _____

_____

I hereby authorize you to release to

_____

_____

any information including the diagnosis and records of any treatment or examination rendered

to me during the period from _____ to _____

_____

SIGNATURE

_____   _____

WITNESS

Figure XII. The standard record release form may be obtained at any business which specializes in office supply. It is important to note that a patient can sign the form and have the records released to themselves.

Occasionally an attorney may send you a written authorization form, signed by the patient, asking you to transfer copies of the records to their office. Comply with their request. The attorney should include a check to cover the administrative costs for this procedure.

WHEN PATIENTS DON'T DO AS REQUESTED

Your records should indicate when a patient does not return for a visit or does not follow a physician or therapist's order as requested. These notations are especially important to an insurance company who needs to know if a patient, insured by their company, is attending therapy as prescribed.

For example, document instances when a patient ambulates to a greater weight bearing than ordered or does an exercise program in a manner other than was instructed. Notations such as these can be invaluable should a patient suffer an adverse result and sue for medical malpractice.

Do not advise a patient on the use of any medication. If the patient appears to be abusing the medication provided, encourage them to contact their doctor or offer to make the phone call for them. Try not to let a patient who may be dangerously overmedicated leave your office. As a professional, you could be partially liable if the patient had an accident. At least encourage them to remain in the office until the effects of the medication have subsided. Do not forceably restrain them.

PROVIDING TESTIMONY

Physical therapists today stand a much greater chance of becoming involved in the legal process of providing testimony than ever before. The profession is growing, as is the public's awareness of the value of therapy and its role in health care.

The legal profession, who at one time sought only the opinion of the physician, is now seeking the physical therapist as an expert in rehabilitation. This professional recognition may be a double-edged sword. It calls for a higher standard of practice by the profession with the greater expectation of "good results" by the public. The expectation of a "good result" could force the practitioner to defend a level of care offered in a malpractice issue. As an expert, the therapist may be forced to justify the quality of care offered.

There are generally three ways that you as a private practitioner may become involved in the legal process of providing testimony. Each way has several unique characteristics which you should be aware of. The three ways are:

1. As a defendant.
2. As a fact witness.
3. As an expert witness.

The legal process is designed to allow opposing sides of a lawsuit a period of time to gather information which may be used to help prove their point of view in court. This period of time which may be as long as several months is called the discovery stage.

The discovery stage is the period of time during the lawsuit when you will be called upon to provide legal testimony. This legal testimony is called a deposition. The deposition is the legal process whereby you give testimony under oath about your knowledge of a particular issue.

You as a Defendant

As a provider of medical care there may be an instance in which a patient alleges you provided medical care which fell below the acceptable standard of care. As a result of this alleged failure to offer acceptable care, the patient may bring a malpractice suit against you alleging that you caused them physical or mental harm.

The most important element of defense to a malpractice case is preparation. From the therapist's standpoint, the preparation begins with contacting your malpractice insurance carrier and arranging a meeting with the lawyer who will provide your defense.

It is essential that you have confidence in the attorney who is assigned to you. You must be able to talk openly with this individual. Set aside enough time to meet with your attorney to explain the treatment you offered, the tests you provided, and the area in which you are accused of wrong doing. In almost all cases, it is your responsibility to provide any medical texts, journals, and illustrations to explain and substantiate your position.

Be straight forward about the treatment you provided to the patient. If there is some area of your involvement which could be questionable, share this information with your attorney. All legal surprises can be avoided through a close working relationship between you and your attorney.

Discuss with your attorney the possibility of retaining experts in the area of question. Consider requesting a former instructor to testify on your behalf as to the standard of care concerning the incident in question. Allow your attorney to confer with any experts you suggest. Your deposition should be taken only after you are convinced that your attorney understands all the issues and is properly prepared.

The Deposition

Make an effort to become involved in all aspects of the malpractice case against you. Do not sit idly without any involvement in the pretrial proceedings. You have the right to sit in on any depositions given by the plaintiff, a witness, or any others who may be involved in the case.

Your involvement in the case can be essential to the final outcome. You can aid your attorney by providing a direction for inquiry. This also gives you an opportunity to observe the plaintiff's attorney. By observing the plaintiff's attorney, you can become acquainted with the style and the attitude that will be directed toward you.

The rules governing a deposition allow the plaintiff's lawyer to ask a wide variety of questions regarding your knowledge, education, skill, and your ability to withstand the questioning in a court room environment. The plaintiff's attorney is going to strongly attempt to obtain evidence favorable to his/her client.

In some cases a skillful attorney will suggest that you may have made changes to records or even suggest your recollection is not proper. At other times you may be asked the same question but in two different ways. This is an attempt to determine your credibility. It is imperative that your attorney prepare you for the types of questions you may be asked.

When testifying, either at the deposition or in court, it is essential that you be truthful, accurate, and straight forward. Following these steps does not, however, guarantee you will be dealt with in a fair way. You will be thoroughly questioned by the plaintiff's attorney who will emphasize only the strong points of his case. Many of your statements may be taken out of context. Any charting errors you made will be brought out in court in an attempt to ridicule your care and the attention given to the patient. There will also be an attempt to suggest you are not telling the truth or attempting to cover up some important detail.

When preparing to give testimony, it is essential you remain as detached as possible. Many times, before the deposition or court room proceedings begin, opposing attorneys engage in friendly conversation about a variety of subjects unrelated to your case. This process can be very misleading and will generally change once the legal proceedings begin. Do not allow yourself to be caught off guard. Try to adopt the attitude that you might use towards an unfriendly or hostile patient.

Do not volunteer any information that is not requested. There are some questions which should be answered with a simple yes or no. As a general rule, only elaborate if your simple answer can, in some way, be taken out of context. If you do not understand the question posed by the attorney, ask that it be repeated or rephrased. If a question is extremely broad or misleading, do not try to specifically answer it. Think slowly, take your time and give a complete answer.

It is also perfectly acceptable for you to forget some item relative to the patient's treatment. There are times when certain details cannot be recalled. Do not answer a question on an assumption. It is much better to simply say, "I cannot remember."

Another misunderstanding relevent to providing testimony is that once an answer is given it cannot be corrected. This is not true. Once you realize you have made an incorrect statement, it is perfectly acceptable to state that you had something else in mind or did not understand the question. Then give the correct response.

Try to remain confident and optimistic. Very few attorneys will be as well prepared for all the medical issues as you are. If you are well versed in the legal process and the issues concerning the case, the deposition will not be a traumatic event. Presenting yourself as a well trained, highly qualified and believable witness can be an important factor in the plaintiff's attorney's willingness to pursue the case. The deposition is the testing ground where the defendant's trial capabilities are evaluated. The amount of preparation put into your deposition will have a significant impact on the final disposition of the lawsuit.

The Physical Therapist as a Defendant: A seventy-five-year-old male with a history of a stroke and right side hemiparesis was referred to a private practitioner for gait training. He presented a history of numerous falls due to poor balance. While gait training at the facility, the patient lost his balance and fell, fracturing his left hip. After being discharged from the hospital, the patient spent four weeks in an extended care facility.

The patient sued the private practitioner for negligent health care. Evidence was presented which indicated there was no safety belt on the man at the time of the fall. The plaintiff's attorney successfully argued that had a safety belt been in place, the impact of the fall could have been lessened if not prevented entirely. The plaintiff was awarded one hundred and thirty eight thousand dollars.

Fact Witness

As a fact witness you will be asked to simply summerize the treatment you provided to a patient. This may be nothing more than to explain the physical condition of the patient at the time of discharge.

If you are called as a fact witness, you must determine if there is a potential of becoming a defendant. An attorney may have the intent of asking you to testify, as an unrepresented party, and then use your sworn testimony against you in a medical malpractice case. If this possibility seems likely, you must notify your insurance carrier so they can provide an attorney at the deposition.

The Physical Therapist as a Fact Witness: An eighty-two-year-old female with marked osteoporosis suffered a severe fracture of the right shoulder after slipping on an unmarked wet surface in a local restaurant. The shoulder required surgery to reduce the fracture as well as extensive therapy.

The issue in court was not whether the restaurant was negligent, that was quite evident. The primary area of concern involved the amount of monetary damages to be awarded for loss of functional use of the extremity. The plaintiff's attorney argued the woman would remain in constant pain and have only limited use of the extremity.

To help prove the case, the attorney questioned the physical therapist who provided rehabilitation. The therapist summarized objective findings and concluded that additional range of motion could not be obtained and that functional movement would be limited. The plaintiff prevailed in the case.

Hypothetical Expert Witness

As a physical therapist, you may be called to offer testimony concerning the standard of care in a case. The plaintiff and defendant may be unknown to you. You will be asked to review a medical record and determine if the care that the patient received met the generally accepted standard of care in physical therapy. In this case, you will be considered an expert in the area which is being examined. You will be questioned as to what you would do under "hypothetically" similar circumstances. Before agreeing to be an expert witness, examine your background and training in the area of legal interest. For example, if your professional career has primarily been concerned with treating orthopaedic patients, do not offer your expert opinion in a matter involving pediatrics.

The Physical Therapist as an Expert Witness: A sixty-one-year-old male auto mechanic sustained an above the knee amputation as a result of a truck slipping off a hydraulic lift. In an effort to prove damages, the plaintiff's attorney wanted to establish whether ambulation and the ability to retain a job would become more difficult as the man got older.

The attorney contacted a physical therapist who was able to provide him with several research studies documenting the increased energy expenditure required for both above and below knee amputees. Research also indicated that elderly individuals have an increased chance of falling over small objects and greater difficulty regaining their balance after starting to fall. The information provided by the physical therapist allowed the attorney to successfully present the case.

THE USE OF AUTHORITATIVE LITERATURE

When an attorney cites a particular author, journal article, or book, beware. If you concede that a given individual or article is authoritative, it may be taken as "gospel." Once designated as such, it may be used against you in court.

There is no strict definition of the word "authoritative." If you do not want to be impeached with authoritative literature you must point out that you either agree or disagree with many of the items contained in the publication, but that overall, you do not accept it as authoritative.

If the attorney then attempts to read you portions of the publication, do not offer an opinion on what is read. To prevent being taken out of context, ask for sufficient time to read the entire publication.

Do not comment on general areas of medicine for which you do not have sufficient training. Attorneys may ask you to offer an opinion as to "what you feel was wrong with the patient." After carefully listening to your reply they may quickly point out that you lack the proper training to "diagnose an illness." This could strongly discredit your overall testimony and weaken the case.

Be aware of certain key words which can be used by an attorney to imply much more than what you meant. Words such as "usually" or "routinely" may seem innocent but may be used in court to mean that to do otherwise would fall below the standard of care and subsequently be negligent.

PROPERLY DISCHARGING A PATIENT

There are guidelines to follow to properly discharge a patient from under physical therapy care. Once you, as a private practitioner, offer to treat a patient you are generally obligated to continue to provide treatment. The patient/physical therapist relationship, once initiated, continues until one of the following occurs:

1. It is ended by the parties' mutual consent.
2. It is revoked by the patient.
3. The therapist's services are no longer needed.
4. The therapist withdraws from the case after reasonable notice to the patient.

As a private practitioner following these guidelines, it often becomes very difficult to schedule any leisure time away from the practice for vacations and/or medical conferences. There is always one patient who needs physical therapy and cannot be discharged from under your care. Many practitioners follow the example of the medical profession and obtain another local physical therapist to see their patients while they are out of town. Various compensation agreements can be worked out for such coverage between practitioners.

What Constitutes Improper Discharge of a Patient?

The legal profession uses the word "abandonment" to denote the improper discharge of a patient. It is essential that you be aware of what constitutes abandonment so you can avoid any potential difficulties. The following areas would constitute abandonment by the physical therapist.

1. **Express withdrawal.** Asking a patient to leave your facility without legal justification. (Example: Asking a patient, who you are presently treating, not to return to your facility because the physical therapy bill has not been paid.)

2. **Premature discharge of a patient.** (Example: Having a patient follow a home program without maintaining a periodic check on their progress. Because of this, the patient's condition deteriorated, requiring additional medical care to correct the problem.)

3. **Failure to instruct the patient adequately.** (Example: Apparently poor gait training resulted in a fall, causing further injury to the patient.)

Defenses to "Abandonment"

There is a legal recourse which may be assumed as a defense to allegations that you did not properly discharge a patient. It is important to keep in mind that all patients you plan to discharge must be given sufficient notice so if they wish, they can secure another provider of physical therapy.

The defenses to abandonment are:

1. Designation of a qualified substitute physical therapist.
2. Unreasonable demands made by a patient.
3. Lack of cooperation by a patient.

Physical therapists occasionally treat a patient who, for whatever reason, can no longer be helped by further treatment. Keeping in mind the possible need for future documentation in difficult cases, you would be advised to communicate your final position in writing and have it delivered by certified mail.

Mrs. XXXX
XXX Florida Avenue
Anytown, Florida

December 31, 19XX

Dear Mrs. XXXX:

Due to repeated failures to attend the scheduled physical therapy appointments, I am unable to schedule any further physical therapy appointments at this time. Each time a physical therapy appointment is scheduled I receive either last minute notice or no notice at all of your inability to attend. Other patients would like to receive physical therapy during that time period but are unable to because it is filled.

There are currently two other physical therapy centers within a short distance of this location. They are:

1. Anywhere Physical Therapy   Phone: 727-XXXX

2. Anyplace Physical Therapy   Phone: 727-XXXO

Upon your written request, I will gladly forward all records concerning your treatment to the chosen facility. Enclosed is the referral as provided by your physician.

Sincerely,

XXXX, R.P.T.

Figure XIII. A certified letter such as this protects you against a patient who may become hostile and claim they were abandoned. This letter supplies a qualified substitute, demonstrates the patient's lack of cooperation, and provides them with a referral to lessen the length of time they may have to wait for therapy while seeking another referral from their physician.

CHAPTER SIX

PURCHASING OR BUILDING A FACILITY

EVERY physical therapist would like to design a private practice that is very cost effective. Many questions enter your mind when you begin to plan a facility. Questions such as how to determine how much space is needed in a practice to offer the best quality medical care? What is the best floor plan for a practice? How do you decide on the type of construction? It is important, however, to thoroughly examine all questions which arise. Errors in practice design, once overlooked, can be very expensive to correct.

Consider your present employment situation. Are the doorways wide enough to be wheelchair accessible? How wide should a doorway be in order to accommodate a wheelchair? Is there sufficient seating space for all patients in the waiting room? Does the staff have an area away from patients where they can write chart notes or take a lunch break?

These questions, as well as many others, are often overlooked by the beginning private practitioner. They are overlooked simply because the physical therapist is not trained to examine questions such as these. Professional training cannot cover every aspect of the business world. Due to the vast amount of medical education which must be covered in only a few short years, the medical profession (physical therapists, doctors, and dentists) cannot be schooled in all aspects of private practice and facility planning.

There are no complete answers to planning a facility. Your goal should be to develop and answer as many questions as possible about your practice interests and professional aspirations. This should be done long before beginning to plan or construct a facility. This chapter discusses some of the many factors which must be considered when purchasing or building a facility. It is essential to consider all available

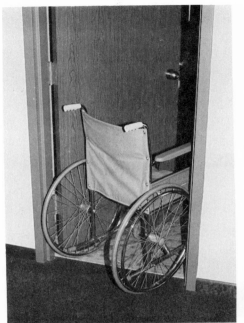 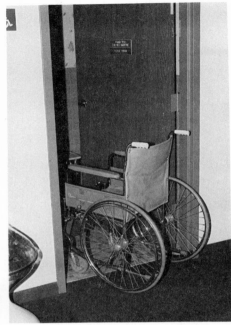

Figure XIV. Doorways should be a minimum of thirty six inches wide. These photographs demonstrate the problems encountered when entrances are too small. Also include handrails to assist in transfers.

options before deciding on a course of action. A well planned facility is essential to providing a good management environment and a successful practice.

WHERE TO BEGIN

Before you can consider purchasing or building a facility you must examine your long-term goals. Will the practice be as an individual, group, or as a partnership? Each option has advantages and disadvantages which must be considered prior to choosing a course of action. If you decide to recruit one or more partners, the space requirements of the practice may change. Each partner may desire or need an individual office. Any proposed construction must examine the possibility of practice expansion.

As the practice begins to grow you may need to hire additional office personnel. A growing practice will probably require more floor space for the waiting room as well as for patient treatment. As a business person, you cannot afford to change locations every four to five years simply to keep up with practice growth. Keep in mind, you are planning not just for now but for the future. To have a successful private practice requires long-term planning. To plan for the long term means to plan five years in advance.

THE CHOICE OF A FACILITY

Areas of high growth, both now and in the future, are some of the best locations for establishing a practice. If you are considering a specific community, there must be a careful examination of the long-term aspects for the surrounding area. Areas of a city which offer office space at below market rates may be in the process of decline. These same areas may have older office buildings which, although well constructed, may be difficult to remodel or expand. Parking in older areas of a city may also be difficult. Survey the proposed location to determine how far a person with ambulation difficulties would have to walk to reach the facility from the nearest parking area.

If you decide to locate in a city, consider attempting to establish the practice as close to the university medical center or hospital as possible. These areas tend to draw a larger population base and are frequently provided with a public transportation system. In areas where parking space is limited, the population may rely heavily on public transportation to reach the practice location.

ONCE YOU FIND A LOCATION: PURCHASING A BUILDING

The ideal practice situation for many physical therapists is to own their own facility. Owning a facility can be an excellent investment depending on the real estate under consideration. Before purchasing any commercial structure, have it surveyed by a professional building inspector. The professional building inspector's job is to closely examine all aspects of the building to determine if it is safe and in working order. A typical inspection will include checks of the plumbing, electrical system, foundation, roof, landscaping, the heating and cooling system, and any appliances which are to be provided.

The individual who will be conducting the inspection of the building will be working for you. This person will be paid by the prospective owner for an unbiased opinion. Fees for this service will vary depending upon the size of the building to be evaluated. In many cases, the inspection can save you thousands of dollars on repairs which you, as an untrained individual, could easily overlook.

The use of a building inspector has many advantages. First of all, the evaluation is an independent examination which is neither influenced by the real estate agent or the seller. A second advantage is that it gives you, as the potential owner of the building, leverage over the seller in the event that something is in need of repair. If the building inspector locates a problem, the buyer can negotiate the purchase price downward, offer to split the repairs, or back out of the deal completely if the problem is serious enough.

The third advantage is the inspection will educate you as the buyer. Most inspectors encourage the prospective buyer to attend the inspection. It will allow you to plan for the financial outlays which may be encountered in the future.

BUILDING AN OFFICE

The decision to construct a new office building will set in motion a series of events. Each of these events will be necessary to ensure the successful construction of a private office. The first step to building a new office is the acquisition of commercial property. This can sometimes be a difficult step since it requires considerable planning and foresight in order to select the appropriate location.

Commercial property can be very expensive to purchase. In many cases, due to the large expenditures for land, the physical therapist must locate and purchase commercial property years before beginning construction. This is because commercial loan agreements often stipulate a fifteen to thirty percent down payment to become eligible for a loan. Requiring steep down payments for loan approval will often cut deep into personal savings. Depending on the size of the down payment, it may take years before the therapist is eligible to finance new building construction. Because of this, the practitioner must purchase land with some expectation as to what the community will be like once financially prepared to build.

THE STEPS OF BUILDING CONSTRUCTION

In the construction of a commercial building you will require the assistance of many individuals. You will need a banker for loan approval, an architect and engineer for building design, and at least one licensed building contractor for construction. To properly visualize the construction process, think of the building as going through four steps.

Step One

Step one involves having the preliminary plans drawn up for your location. The preliminary plans should include all aspects of the building, including the parking lot, the approximate size of each room in the building, the proposed building materials, and a general budget outlining the costs of the project.

Step Two

During this phase you will be presented a more detailed cost estimate for the project. You will be involved in the selection of many of the materials which will be used to construct the facility.

Step Three

Negotiations will begin with a number of contractors who will want to bid on the project. The architect selected should actively engage in all negotiations. It will be the architect's job to guide the practitioner in the proper evaluation and selection of construction bids.

Step Four

Construction of the building begins. During step four you will be expected to make periodic payments to the contractors to allow them to complete construction. Also during this phase, it is essential that you and the architect monitor the progress of construction. If you see potential problems in building construction, have them brought to the attention of the architect. The architect should be responsible for contacting the appropriate individuals to ensure the correction of any construction problems.

IMPORTANT DETAILS

Before undertaking the very expensive process of having an architect draw the preliminary plans for a building, make a rough sketch of your own ideas. The sketch should include an estimate of the square footage requirements. Making a rough sketch will give the architect some direction concerning your construction interests and needs.

Estimate the amount of attic space you would like to have. Many times, outdated equipment and medical records cannot be stored in an office due to insufficient storage space. Consider including either a large attic or basement which can be transformed into a storage area. Allow for proper ventilation in these areas so the effects of heat and humidity do not destroy what is being stored.

For planning purposes, you may want to mark off areas in your living room to simulate the office space requirements. It is generally best to make all estimations a little too large. As the practice grows, you may need the extra office space. Keep in mind, you may someday be interested in selling the practice. What may be just right for you may be too small for someone looking to purchase the practice.

After the preliminary drawings have been made, you will be presented with a projected cost estimate. This estimate will probably rise as the end of construction nears. Make sure it is as realistic as possible so you can budget funds appropriately.

EVALUATING LAND AND POSITIONING THE BUILDING

The more level the property, the less expensive it will be to construct a building and parking lot. Before investing in commercial property, have the land under consideration surveyed to determine the size of the facility which could be constructed. The size of the lot needed to construct a facility is in part determined by the size of the proposed project. There are no general rules to follow. For example, zoning laws in a proposed location may require the commercial structure be a certain distance from the street. This requirement or "set back" can greatly reduce the size of a proposed facility.

Purchasing land which has not been cleared of underbrush and trees is often less expensive. If you do not have immediate construction plans, this may be the best option. Many municipalities require land to be kept mowed once it has been cleared. To avoid monthly mowing charges, check with the city authorities before having the land cleared.

Closely examine the elevation and slope of the property under consideration. If the slope of the property is too steep, it may be difficult for the patients to ambulate. Elderly individuals, who are dependent on walkers and wheelchairs, are very hesitant to attempt ambulation on sloped surfaces. Make every effort to have the parking area and the building on the same level surface.

When purchasing undeveloped property, consult the local zoning authority on landscaping requirements. For example, in some municipalities, each tree cut down to erect a new building must be replaced by two others at the end of construction. Plan the design of the building to accommodate as much of the existing landscape as possible. Large trees can reduce air conditioning costs while at the same time reduce cold winds during winter months.

Give careful consideration to the direction the building will face. Building position is most often influenced by the climate of the region. In northern states, a building which has a front door facing the cold north wind may be inaccessible if it is snowing. A building, on the other hand, which faces east is often provided with ample sunlight in the waiting room. This can help reduce the electrical requirements for lighting. The choice of a direction to position the building should be made with the objective of reducing costs and providing for year around safe usage.

FINANCING BUILDING CONSTRUCTION AND EQUIPMENT

After careful examination of your financial portfolio, a commercial bank may agree to lend you money to construct an office building. If they hesitate, consider using other sources of financial help such as a savings and loan, private investors, and finance companies. The more community minded the commercial bank or savings and loan, the better the chances of obtaining a loan. All banks must follow federal and state regulations, but an individually owned bank may be more receptive to loaning money than an established corporate lending institution.

Always shop around for the best mortgage and interest rate. When possible, obtain a fixed rate mortgage. Have a thorough understanding of any penalties associated with early retirement of a loan. The lending institution should not penalize the practitioner if the loan is paid off early.

Requirements for loan approval will vary. Some lending agencies require property costs not to exceed one-third of the total projected cost. Others specify the land to be paid for before making an application for a mortgage. If presented with an opportunity to purchase land without sufficient time to investigate lending requirements, consider using a real estate option. By using this option you are assured that the location will not be sold during a specified period of time. This will allow you the opportunity to investigate the surrounding community and the various mortgage requirements without binding you to the purchase of the property. Talk with the real estate agent about the advantages and disadvantages of a real estate option.

Be as creative as possible in obtaining your medical equipment. The medical equipment supply business is very competitive. Do not hesitate to negotiate the best deal. Very often you can get an equipment sales company to help finance part of your equipment. Others will allow you to lease the equipment on a monthly basis with an option to buy at the end of the lease.

Avoid ordering equipment prematurely. In some cases, the equipment arrives before construction of the building is complete. You must then pay to have the equipment stored until the building is ready for occupancy. Specify delivery dates only when occupancy is assured.

PLANNING PARKING SPACE REQUIREMENTS

There are several methods for determining the size lot needed and the appropriate parking space requirements. One of the most simple methods is to consider the needs of the anticipated patient load. Elderly individuals, for example, require more area to safely get in and out of cars with walkers or wheelchairs than the average medical office. To plan the parking space requirements, you must determine the maximum patient load the practice could be expected to treat in a one hour period of time.

For example, a physical therapist with two employees may expect to see a maximum number of four patients per hour. The practitioner hopes to run on time but believes no patients will be expected to wait more than fifteen minutes. To accommodate both staff and patients, the therapist would need a minimum of seven parking spaces. If the practice grows and it is decided to bring in another physical therapist and two more employees, the present parking situation would rapidly become

PARKING

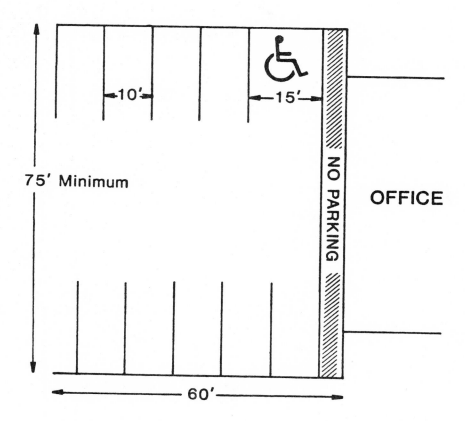

4500 Sq. Ft. Perpendicular − 1 Way

Figure XV. Although parking plans vary, the following demonstrates a possible guideline to planning parking requirements. One space has been provided for handicapped parking.

too small. Keep in mind that even the smallest of cars will require a parking area of at least 9′ × 20′ or one hundred and eighty square feet. Depending on the projected growth of the practice, you may require as much as four times the size of the building for parking.

Corner lots are ideal for maximum exposure and ease of parking. When located near hospitals or medical centers, corner lots will be very expensive. Corner lots in prime areas (150′ × 200′) may have an asking price in excess of $200,000. Property assessment taxes on land such as this can also be very high.

In some municipalities, the zoning commission may require one parking space for every one hundred to two hundred square feet of office space. A practitioner who is planning to construct an office which has a total of eighteen hundred square feet of working space would require a minimum of nine to a maximum of eighteen parking spaces. If each parking space were to measure 11′ × 24′ or two hundred and sixty four square feet each, the practitioner would need a parking area of at least two thousand six hundred and forty square feet to park only ten automobiles. Remember, provisions must also be made for automobiles to turn around in the parking lot.

One area which is frequently overlooked when planning parking is the allowance for service and delivery vehicle space. Design the driveway to be wide enough to help prevent autos and service trucks from driving over landscaping.

In some areas the hospital and the surrounding community may be growing so rapidly that older homes, once only residential, may be re-zoned to commercial structures. Depending on the parking space available, many of those older homes can be purchased for a much lower price than it would cost to build a new structure.

The costs of a paved parking surface will vary depending upon what must be done to prepare the area to be surfaced. Investigate the cost of a concrete parking lot versus a tar surface. Depending upon the climate of the area, one has advantages over the other. Your architect and the local zoning board will be of assistance in selecting the proper surface.

YOUR NEW BUILDING:
CHOOSING YOUR CONSTRUCTION MATERIALS

There are two types of building materials you will be required to evaluate prior to the building of a new office. These are interior materials and exterior materials. Your involvement in the selection of these materials is essential to reducing building costs and providing an attractive practice environment.

When an architect designs the proposed structure he will want to know what you have in mind for exterior construction. Building codes often influence what type of material will be required. It is essential, however, that you refrain from the importation of materials from other areas of the country. This only adds to the cost of the structure and does little to increase the overall value of the building. In general, it is always best to choose materials which will help prevent damage in the event of fire. An insurance agent can provide information on which building materials are considered the safest and will reduce insurance premiums.

Plan very carefully the use and replacement of windows. Double-pane windows will greatly reduce electricity costs by providing greater insulation in the winter and summer. The use of tinted glass will reduce glare. Windows should only be placed in rooms where it is essential to view the outside. Windows in treatment rooms are generally not necessary and only add to construction costs.

Always try to select exterior materials which reduce or require little maintenance. Wood is a good exterior surface depending on the climate. In areas of high humidity, wood deteriorates quickly. Wood must be repainted every two to three years to maintain its durability and appearance. Brick and concrete structures are often easier to maintain and can provide excellent insulation.

Interior materials can be very expensive depending upon what is chosen. Once again, building code requirements frequently determine the minimum construction standards. Choose interior materials which are attractive but not overly expensive. Many physical therapy departments simply use dry wall surfaces for the interior of the building. Although it must be painted every two to three years, it is the most cost effective. If a wall must be moved, dry wall is generally the easiest to tear down and replace without excessive costs. Dry wall provides only an average sound proofing but can be covered by wood paneling to increase its soundproof potential and the attractiveness of the office.

HEATING AND AIR CONDITIONING

The choice of a proper heating and air conditioning unit for your facility is essential. The heating and cooling of an office can be very expensive if too small a unit is installed. Most practitioners, as well as many home owners, choose a forced air system. This is the most economical way to heat or cool an office.

Window unit heating and air conditioning is not very energy efficient. They can be installed easily but do not provide an even cooling or heating of a room. The immediate area around the unit cannot be used because it is either too hot or too cold for patient and employee comfort.

Proper ventilation is becoming increasingly more important to the private practice. Many practitioners are utilizing computers and other electronically sensitive equipment which should not be exposed to high humidity. Make sure there is a system provided to remove humidity quickly from the whirlpool areas. These areas must also be kept dry to prevent growth of bacteria on walls, floors, and equipment.

If you plan to use the attic or basement for storage of old equipment and records, make sure it is properly ventilated. Some practitioners have installed duct work to both heat and cool these areas. As the practice grows, these areas can be partially heated and cooled to maintain the stored contents. Have the architect make provisions in the duct work so as not to cool or heat these areas until needed.

Provisions should also be made for ceiling fan installment. At some point in time the air conditioning may break down requiring several days to repair. If your facility has few windows, ceiling fans can be used to keep the air circulating so as to allow you and the employees to continue seeing patients.

Ask your architect for suggestions about the most cost-effective duct work to circulate both the heating and air conditioning. In all instances, duct work should be well insulated and properly sealed to prevent leaks. Inefficient heating and cooling systems are very expensive to operate. A small leak can greatly increase your monthly electric bills.

THE ELECTRICAL SYSTEM

Physical therapy departments are some of the largest users of electricity. Almost all patient treatment involves the use of electricity. It is extremely important that proper lighting and electrical systems be provided.

The more outlets you plan for the office, the more circuits you should provide in the breaker box. Each circuit can provide electricity to only a certain number of wall outlets. The larger the equipment demands of your facility, the greater the number of circuits which will be required. Consider all the various types of equipment which could be running at one time in the department and plan for future growth and electricity needs.

Electrical wall outlets should be installed approximately five feet apart. This allows equipment to be moved to accommodate for patient treatment. The outlets themselves should be placed twenty four to thirty six inches off the floor. Make sure all of the wall outlets are properly grounded, especially in whirlpool areas.

Overhead fluorescent lighting is best for areas where patient treatments are to be performed. Lighting should provide for equal intensity throughout all treatment areas. In areas where clerical work or patient charting is performed, higher intensity lighting should be provided. In patient waiting rooms, incadescent table or floor lamps are recommended. Keep lamps at equal distances apart for even room lighting.

WATER SYSTEMS AND OFFICE PLUMBING

An average physical therapy department may use well over one thousand gallons of water per day, most of which is for whirlpools. It is therefore essential that an adequate supply of water be provided to prevent waiting for whirlpools to fill.

The larger the diameter of pipe supplying fresh water to your whirlpool area, the faster it can be filled. In some instances, practitioners have overlooked incoming water supply needs and, as a result, had a long period of waiting (ten to fifteen minutes) for a whirlpool to fill.

Proper water removal systems are also essential. Make sure all drains which remove water from your whirlpool are the largest possible size. It is essential that water be removed as quickly as possible so that whirlpools can be refilled for patient treatment. Per average; one hundred gallons of water will take eight to ten minutes to drain with a one to one and a half inch pipe. Depending on your patient volume, too small a drainage system can limit patient treatment potential.

Adequate water heater size is a priority consideration. It may take thirty to forty-five minutes to heat one hundred gallons of water to an acceptable temperature for patient treatment when using an electric water heater. This is entirely too slow if you plan to perform one to two whirlpools per hour. Allow room for the largest available water heater to accommodate your hydro-therapy needs. If gas is available, consider it as an alternative to electricity. Gas water heaters typically heat much faster and are more economical than electric water heating systems.

If you plan a large landscaped area for your office, install a sprinkler system. In most cases it is best to install an electric timer that will automatically water the landscaping. Timers placed on both sprinkler systems and water heating systems can reduce overall electricity costs. If a timer is installed on your water heating system, program it to heat water throughout the day, turn off in the afternoon or early evening, and to come on early the next morning.

Each bathroom and whirlpool fixture should have a shut off valve so any repairs can be made without turning off the entire water supply to the office. Sinks should have wrist controls to allow for easy turn on and off by handicapped individuals. All toilets should be hung from the walls to allow for the ease of underneath cleaning. No carpeting should be installed in any area where there is a large usage of water. Tile covered floors are easily cleaned and promote far less bacterial growth.

If you are considering the rental of an office, examine all existing plumbing. Remember, any major modifications you make to the building to accommodate its plumbing needs will probably accrue to the owner if you decide to leave. Some buildings will require major structural changes if the plumbing system is modified.

Consider the installation of floor drains in areas where patients get out of whirlpools. These floors often get wet and can become very dangerous if not quickly dried. Floor drains will eliminate many standing water problems.

REDUCING NOISE LEVELS

Physical therapists engage in a large number of conversations on subjects which may vary in topic. Some conversations may be private in nature which the patient may not want others to overhear.

To eliminate this problem, choose interior materials which will reduce noise levels and allow for greater privacy. Drapes and rugs in patient treatment areas will reduce noise levels. Employee offices and lounges should be located away from patient treatment areas and properly soundproofed. Sound is easily carried through back to back electrical outlets and plumbing fixtures. Design the office to allow for maximum privacy in patient/therapist conversations as well as employee conversations.

CHOICE OF LANDSCAPING

When planning the landscaping of a building you must take into consideration not only the attractiveness of the plants chosen, but the primary functions they can serve. Landscaping can be an excellent insulator and soundproofing device. Many practitioners simply allow the architect to choose whatever would look best for their location. Others hire a local landscaper to provide the landscaping service at the end of building construction.

Depending on your work schedule, do your own landscape planning and shopping. In most cases you can plant trees and do your own landscaping at up to fifty percent of the cost of a landscaper.

DRAWING YOUR PROPOSED STRUCTURE:
THE WAITING ROOM

The first area of a practice that a patient comes in contact with is the waiting room. This area should be designed so that it presents a pleasant surrounding and provides comfortable seating. All areas of a waiting room should be visable from the receptionist's desk.

THE PATIENT RECEPTION ROOM

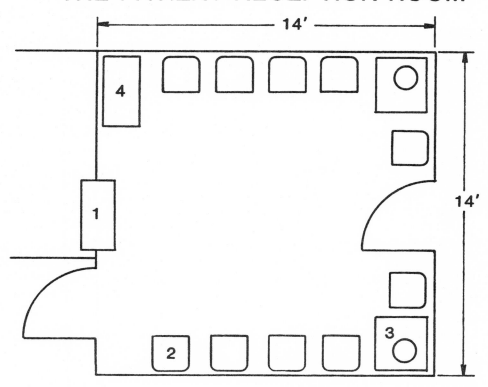

196 square feet
10 seats

1. Receptionist Station
2. Patient Chair
3. End Table & Lamp
4. Magazine Rack

Figure XVI. The reception room should be designed so that patients have few objects to avoid during ambulation. An area should be set aside for wheelchair parking but still allow patients access to all chairs in the reception room.

To increase practice efficiency, some practitioners install a telephone on the wall in the waiting room. The phone is installed so that only local calls can be made. This allows patients to schedule for transportation without tying up the office phones.

Carpeting should be installed in the waiting room to reduce noise levels. It is advisable that all carpeting have a low nap and be durable enough to withstand heavy traffic and avoid wear. Waiting rooms which enter directly from the outside should have water resistant carpeting.

THE BUSINESS OFFICE

The receptionist will be the individual primarily responsible for collecting funds from the patients, typing new charts, and filing charts not currently in use. The business office should provide a comfortable working environment and enhance employee productivity.

It is essential that at least one chair be provided in the business office which will allow a patient to privately discuss his/her bill. If you plan on billing by computer it is best to locate the chair so the receptionist will have easy access to the computer while talking with the patient.

Provide noise protection between the business office and the waiting room by using a soundproof glass. It is important that the receptionist be able to converse on the telephone freely without being overheard by patients in the waiting room. If additional privacy is desired, it may be obtained by the use of opaque glass. In most practice situations it is also recommended that the business office have a clear view of the entire physical therapy department. When this is provided, a receptionist can assess whether patients are receiving treatment on schedule and what changes should be made to improve scheduling efficiency. This arrangement also allows the receptionist to communicate effectively with staff members concerning phone calls.

PATIENT TREATMENT AREAS

The patient treatment areas are where the practitioner will spend most of his/her time in direct contact with patients. It is therefore

THE BUSINESS OFFICE

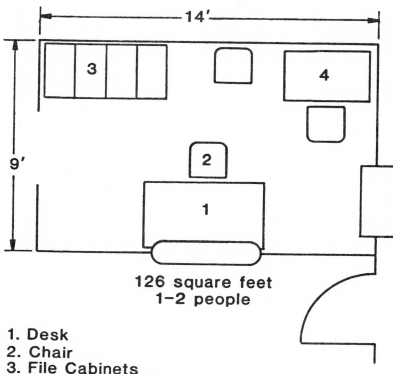

126 square feet
1–2 people

1. Desk
2. Chair
3. File Cabinets
4. Typing Desk/Computer Terminal

Figure XVII. The drawing provides two areas for the receptionist to converse with a patient. The hallway can be used for routine scheduling whereas the business office can be used to discuss more private matters.

essential that these areas be designed to allow for maximum convenience and efficiency. In order to determine how much space is needed for patient treatment you must determine how much space is required for patient care.

As an individual practitioner, plan at least enough space to treat four patients simultaneously. If one or more partners will eventually be joining the practice, allow at least the same amount of room for them. In most practices, you should plan a treatment space of at least eight by ten feet to comfortably accommodate all types of physical therapy treatment.

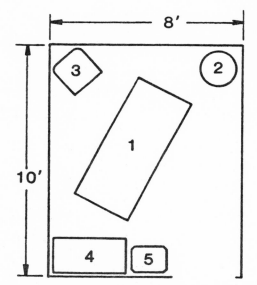

1. Treatment Table
2. Adjustable Stool
3. Chair
4. Linen Cabinet
5. Sink

Figure XVIII. The drawing indicates the treatment room is isolated from the rest of the department by walls. This can be a costly expenditure. As a beginning practitioner you may wish to utilize curtains to provide privacy.

All rooms should be designed to provide for the least amount of walking and equipment movement by the practitioner. The more modalities your practice offers, the greater the space requirements. If possible, plan all treatment rooms identically. This allows you to develop a consistant pattern of movement throughout the office. Over the life of the practice, this will save time. If each room is designed differently, you must constantly adjust your movements. This can become very time consuming and tiresome for the practitioner and the employees.

PRACTICE TIPS

1. Carpet whatever possible. Carpeting promotes quietness and reduces employee fatigue. The use of carpeting also reduces the number and severity of falls.

2. All doorways should be wheelchair accessible.

3. Each treatment room should have a signaling device which will allow either a patient or an employee to signal in the event of an emergency.

4. No patient treatment area should be exposed to a draft. Air conditioning and heating ducts should not face treatment tables.

5. Provide enough room to allow a patient to change clothing. Several clothes hooks should be provided in each room. A mirror may be provided either on the back of the door or on the wall.

6. Areas for note taking should be provided in each patient treatment room. Consider whether you are right or left handed when planning these areas. Writing areas may be at sitting or standing height depending upon your personal preference.

7. Enough space should be provided to allow for a complete opening of all cabinets and drawers. Whenever possible, stock each cabinet and drawer with identical supplies to reduce the time required to locate needed materials.

8. Each area should have sufficient lighting. It is not recommended to use table lamps in patient treatment rooms.

9. Patient restrooms should be separate from employee restrooms. Each patient restroom should be wheelchair accessible and allow enough room for the patient, the wheelchair, and at least one aide. Emergency signals should also be included in patient restrooms. Patient restrooms should not be equipped with locking doors.

10. All cabinets should be at a height which is accessible for shorter employees. Do not choose more cabinets than will be needed. Most medical equipment is unable to be stored inside a typical cabinet space. Allow only enough space for linens and the most frequently required physical therapy equipment.

HYDROTHERAPY

Design of a hydrotherapy department basically follows the same guidelines as were described in designing the patient treatment areas. Allow enough room to comfortably and safely get a patient in and out of a whirlpool. In general, allow an area of about ten feet by eight feet to accommodate a one hundred gallon knee whirlpool. This provides enough room to comfortably change clothes and easily ambulate with an assistive device. Whirlpool areas should be properly ventilated and not carpeted. Heat lamps may be installed in the ceiling to provide additional warmth.

The floor should be either tile or some other nonskid surface which is designed to prevent falls. No patient should be allowed to independently get in or out of a whirlpool. All electrical outlets should be located away from areas where water could be splashed. Patients should be

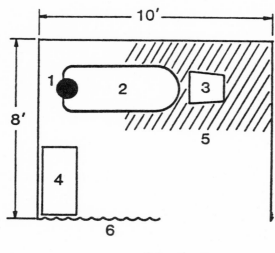

1. Whirlpool Motor
2. Whirlpool
3. Elevated Seat
4. Linens/Supplies
5. Non—Skid Surface
6. Curtain

80 sq. feet

Figure XIX. In most out-patient practices, at least one side of a whirlpool may be located near a wall. This saves space that is generally not needed to provide effective treatment. Remember to provide enough room on all sides so employees can safely assist in patient transfer activities.

discouraged from turning whirlpools on or off. Enough room should also be provided to allow a stretcher to be used in the patient treatment areas.

THE GYM

There are no specific guidelines as to the proper area to set aside in planning for a physical therapy gym. Each practitioner must independently determine equipment needs and the space requirements for proper use of the equipment.

The practitioner should plan enough space so that equipment does not have to be moved to accommodate its full usage in patient treatment areas. Items such as parallel bars must be accessible from at least three sides. Enough space should also be provided to allow equipment to be utilized by wheelchair confined individuals.

When planning the gym, consider future practice growth. In the initial stages of your practice you may not be financially prepared to spend $50,000 to $60,000 on the latest equipment. As the practice grows, plan to set aside areas for the installation of the most modern and frequently used equipment. Equipment should be positioned so that it will be easy to observe all patients from any point in the office.

UTILITY AND STORAGE AREAS

Utility space is typically where the hot water heater and the air conditioner units are stored. These areas should be well vented to prevent over heating and a possible fire. No air conditioning duct should blow air directly on the water heater since this will greatly increase water heating bills.

Many practitioners also allow space for the installation of washers and dryers. Laundry costs can exceed fifty dollars a week in a busy practice. The installation of a washer and dryer can greatly reduce variable costs over the life of the practice. Employees can generally wash laundry throughout the day while still assisting the practitioner in patient treatment. The purchase of commercial laundry equipment is not necessary if the washer and dryer are not overloaded. If you plan to install a dryer make sure provisions are made so the unit can be vented outside.

Storage space is a must in all practices. Do not allow a small closet to become the only storage space when designing the practice facility. Consider what equipment the practice will utilize (splints, canes, athletic tape, etc.) and whether it would be best to have several small closets or one large walk-in closet.

WAITING ROOM FURNITURE

The patient waiting room will be used more than any other room in the office. It is not necessary to consult an interior decorator to design the waiting room or the interior of the office. You can make many of the furniture selections yourself. It is always more costly to have someone design an interior office than it would be for you to do it yourself. The number one rule in interior office design is to never choose any furniture from a picture or catalog unless you have had an opportunity to inspect a floor model first.

There are many grades of furniture to choose from for an office. In most cases it is best to select furniture which is comfortable yet extremely durable. Keep in mind, as many as one to two hundred people a week may sit in one waiting room chair. The furniture must be well built to withstand that type of punishment for a three to five-year period.

Do not purchase a couch for a waiting room. Individual chairs are a better selection. Individual chairs with easy to clean plastic surfaces will last the longest. Depending on the practice, at least 75 percent of your chairs should have individual arm rests. Elderly patients and patients with low back injuries frequently complain that waiting room chairs are either too low or too difficult to get out of once seated. Select a chair which will accommodate the height of an average individual and will give enough support to a person with a low back injury.

Place all chairs either against the wall or back to back. Do not place any chair in the middle of a room where it could tip over backwards. In offices with either wallboard or paneled surfaces consider the installation of chair rails to prevent damage to the interior surfaces.

The number of chairs you will require in the waiting room depends upon the anticipated patient load. To reduce costs, do not buy more chairs than needed simply to fill a waiting room. Per chair costs may be as much as two hundred dollars. As long as you do not buy dealer closeouts, you can always add chairs as the practice expands.

If you permit smoking, keep in mind it will reduce the longevity of both the carpet and furniture installed. Smoke dulls surfaces and creates an odor which clings to fabrics. Post clearly marked "smoking prohibited" signs on at least two walls in the waiting room and enforce the policy.

If you provide music in the waiting room, do not place the stereo receiver where it can be adjusted by the patients. Place the unit in the receptionist's area so the station selection and volume can be maintained at comfortable levels for employees and patients.

All waiting rooms should provide reading material. Place reading material in plastic covers to maintain its attractiveness. Make sure all materials are clearly marked with the name of your office. Choose reading materials which would be of interest to the majority of patients in your practice. Do not allow magazines to become outdated or to be removed from the office by patients or staff members. As a rule, no magazine should be left in the waiting room for a period greater than four to six months.

If your practice will have a large number of children in the waiting room it is best to provide a small table and chairs as well as some books to keep them occupied. You may also consider installing a drinking fountain and a bathroom within close proximity to the waiting room. Encourage the receptionist to closely watch all children left in the waiting room by parents. Also establish a policy that children be disciplined as necessary.

RECEPTIONIST OFFICE FURNITURE AND SUPPLIES

Sufficient counter space must be provided for the receptionist. Counter space should allow at least enough room for a typewriter, calculator, personal computer, and the dictating equipment. Phones should be mounted on the wall to provide the receptionist with a larger working area.

Provide one chair for each person working in the receptionist's office. Chairs should be the swivel type for easy movement. Arm rests on the chairs are optional and should only be provided upon individual request.

All office equipment purchased should include a demonstration by the sales person as to how to properly use and maintain the equipment. Almost all office supply equipment manufacturers provide service contracts on their equipment. The contracts can be very expensive and may cover only a few of the items which may need repair. Read all service contracts thoroughly before agreeing to purchase. Many companies provide a thirty-day trial period on all equipment before the service contract takes effect. If so, wait the thirty days and then purchase the contract if you decide the equipment sufficiently meets your needs.

CHOICE OF OFFICE COLORS

The proper choice of colors for your practice is essential. Color choices should be determined in part by the age of the patient load and by your own personal preferences. Colors create emotions. Bright colors may be too intense and hard on the eyes. Light browns are often perceived as very warm colors. They, like light blues, can be very relaxing to a nervous patient. The use of these colors may help to reduce tension and anxiety.

Green can produce an outdoors effect. Combined with live or artificial plants, it can produce a colorful environment for an office. White should be avoided since it creates an atmosphere similar to a hospital setting. Off-white, however, can be very attractive when combined with browns and beiges.

Solid color wall to wall carpeting generally makes a room look much larger. Solid color carpeting should not, however, be too dark since it shows wear and lint more easily. Shag carpeting should be avoided since it is unsafe when combined with walkers and crutches.

CHAPTER SEVEN

THE DAILY OPERATIONS
OF THE PRACTICE

HOW PATIENTS are treated by staff members is one of the most critical, but often ignored, areas of private practice. Many excellent private practitioners have had long established patient and professional rapport ruined by an inappropriate attitude or action of a staff member. The office personnel, often with the best of intentions, screen phone calls and attempt to lessen some of the daily distractions. In the process, however, patients sometimes become offended by the way their questions and problems are handled. Many patients never openly express their dissatisfaction but instead privately vow never to return to the practice.

This chapter discusses how to properly manage the daily operations of a practice. Each staff member must be trained in the proper techniques for handling all potential patient contracts. At all times, even under the worst of circumstances, the staff members must remain calm and polite. As the owner of the practice, it is your responsibility to establish guidelines for proper employee behavior.

COMMUNICATING THE PRACTICE PHILOSOPHY
OVER THE TELEPHONE: THE ROLE
OF THE RECEPTIONIST

The telephone is a vital part of any private practice. How the phone is answered will quite often determine a patient's willingness to seek out the services offered by the practitioner. It is essential that courtesy characterize every telephone conversation and patient contact. The individual who answers the phone must project a positive image of the physical therapists and staff who work at the facility.

For many patients, the receptionist is the first person encountered in the practice. How a patient is greeted, either by telephone or in person will often determine a patient's outlook towards the practice. In most cases a patient will leave a practice, not due to a poor quality of care, but due to a staff discourtesy.

Each time the receptionist answers the phone, he or she will be confronted with a new situation. Encourage the receptionist to listen carefully without interrupting. It is essential that no patient be left with the feeling that "they just don't seem to have enough time to listen to my problem." All conversations must communicate a genuine interest in a patient's well-being.

The choice of words used by the receptionist is also very important. The receptionist should not say, "Ms. Smith, the physical therapist cannot come to the phone right now." This may accurately describe the situation but unfortunately lead the patient to believe that their question or concern is not important. It is more acceptable to say, "I'm sorry, the therapist is working with a patient at the moment and is unable to come to the phone. Could I take a message or have her return your call?" In any situation where the patient's immediate request cannot be met, assure them it will be handled as soon as possible.

Whenever a patient presents a complaint either in person or by telephone, encourage the receptionist to listen to the entire story. If the receptionist is confronted by a loud or hostile patient, request that the receptionist not react in a like manner. The louder the patient becomes, the more serene the employee should remain. Encourage the receptionist to have the patient offer potential solutions to the problem. In all situations try to calm the patient, either before they leave the office or end the telephone conversation.

In physical therapy, it is quite common for patients to discuss their disabilities with one another while in the waiting room or the same treatment area. Do not allow the receptionist, or any other staff member to discuss a patient's case with another patient. Each patient has a legal right to privacy. Staff members should never disclose any information about a patient via the telephone or with another individual without the express written permission of the patient.

In some instances, the private practitioner may start out without the assistance of a full-time receptionist. Do not, however, leave a waiting

THE TELEPHONE MESSAGE SYSTEM

To:	Date:
From:	Time:
Phone Number	Ext.
Message	

	Phoned		Will Call Again
	Returned Call		Urgent
	Please Call		New Patient
	Was In		Est. Patient
SIGNED:			

Figure XX. Use a message pad which provides a carbon copy of all messages. The copy should become part of the patient's permanent record.

room unattended without providing some means of allowing a patient to let you know that they have arrived. In practice situations such as these it is perfectly acceptable to post a sign which requests the patients register their name and ring a bell before being seated.

SCHEDULING PATIENT APPOINTMENTS

Appointment scheduling is the art of matching the physical therapist and staff members time with the time available for patient treatment. The more efficiently patients are scheduled, the more time will be available for each patient treatment.

Patients are sensitive to the amount of time that is spent with them. It is not uncommon for a patient to note the time spent working with them in comparison to the time spent in the waiting room. Patients do not like to be kept waiting. If they are on time they expect the courtesy to be returned to them by the practitioner. Patients will understand an occasional fifteen-minute delay as long as it is not a common occurance.

Good patient scheduling has two purposes. The first is to maximize the therapist's and staff members' time so there is a consistant flow of patients for treatment. The second is to reduce the amount of time the patient spends in the waiting room or in a treatment area.

A smooth running private practice is established through proper scheduling. Proper scheduling reduces the chances of error and creates a more comfortable practice environment. Although there are many symptoms of poor scheduling, the three most common are:

1. Patient complaints about long waiting periods or rushed treatment times.
2. A large number of patients who do not show up for appointments or cancel at the last moment.
3. The therapist and staff feeling over worked or disorganized at the end of each working day.

EFFICIENT PATIENT SCHEDULING

Good small business management calls for the efficient use of practitioner time in the treatment of patients. A private practice in physical therapy will operate the most efficiently if all patients are seen only by appointment.

Setting up a practice on the appointment basis works well as long as patients arrive on time. Setting aside the appropriate amount of time most often depends on the disability presented by the patient and the specialities of treatment provided by the practice. The following provides suggestions to use in developing a well organized patient appointment system.

1. **Arrive early.** All members of the practice, including the practitioner, should arrive fifteen to twenty minutes before the first scheduled patient appointment. This will assure that operations start on time and help minimize the chances of falling behind.

2. **Plan the treatment flow.** Try to minimize the length of time any one patient must spend waiting for treatment. For example, try to allot sufficient time for a patient receiving a whirlpool to move directly to the exercise equipment without waiting for another patient to finish treatment.

3. **Avoid Walk-Ins.** One thing which will quickly anger a patient is to see someone else taken ahead of them. In most practice situations this is relatively simple to avoid. There are, however, situations which will demand immediate attention.

As a member of the medical profession you will occasionally receive requests from other providers of health care to see a patient as soon as possible. A medical doctor, for example, may request a patient be seen "as soon as possible to prevent the deterioration of a condition."

Some patient problems do require immediate attention. Each practitioner must be prepared to set aside a period during the business day in which a patient, requiring immediate treatment, can be worked in. In many cases you will only be able to spend a few moments with the patient. At least attempt to see the individual and then schedule them for the following business day.

Practitioners often recommend that those patients who must be worked in be seen at the end of the day. Patients without scheduled appointments are generally willing to take whatever time is available. Putting work-in patients at the end of the day will prevent other patients from encountering long waiting periods.

4. **When a patient calls for an appointment, be prepared to ask the proper questions and provide the necessary information.** Encourage the receptionist to be prepared to discuss the insurance information required, fees, and information needed for proper scheduling. If possible, obtain the patient's current address and offer to send them a copy of the practices information brochure. Preparing patients for the first treatment session decreases the likelihood of no-shows and improves office efficiency.

5. **Design your practice appointment book.** Depending on the size of the practice, the number of patients treated, and the type of rehabilitation provided you may need several appointment books. Office supply stores often have a wide variety of small business appointment books for the medical and nonmedical businesses. Some of these books may sufficiently meet your needs. If they are unable to provide one to meet your practice requirements then design one to your liking and have it printed.

6. **Follow the schedule.** Patients who arrive early for appointments should not be seen ahead of those who arrive on time. When a patient arrives ahead of schedule, advise them that another patient will be in soon and that you will see them as soon as possible.

7. **Plan for absences.** An appointment book should always include enough room to indicate when practice members will be absent for vacations or to attend meetings. No patient should arrive to find their appointment suddenly cancelled because of an unexpected meeting which had not been recorded in the appointment book.

8. **Calling patients back.** As a small business owner you will soon notice that the practice receives a large number of telephone calls. You

cannot stop each patient treatment to answer the volume of questions sometimes received during a normal business day. Each telephone call must be evaluated concerning the need for immediate attention.

One of the most important functions your receptionist will perform is to properly screen patient telephone calls. The receptionist should try to determine the purpose of each call and if it can be handled without involving the practitioner. When it is essential to talk on the phone during office hours the practitioner should keep the conversation as brief as possible. Even if the conversation is with a physician, avoid small talk. Remember, there is a patient who is awaiting your return.

The practitioner must attempt to return telephone calls during the same day they are received. Try to set aside a specific time during the business day to return telephone calls. Have the receptionist record the reason you are to return the call as well as advising the individual the approximate time you will be contacting them.

METHODS FOR SCHEDULING PATIENTS

There are many methods available to use in scheduling patients. Each has its advantages and disadvantages depending on the type of rehabilitation to be provided. The following methods are some of the most common in private practice.

Individual or Sequential Scheduling

One of the most popular types of patient scheduling is where each patient is assigned a specific appointment time. In utilizing this method a patient is scheduled every few minutes. At fifteen minute intervals, for example, the first patient will be seen as 8:00 A.M., the second at 8:15 A.M., and so forth. This can be a very complex scheduling system since some patients will require only a few minutes while others, such as new patients, will require more time. When it can be determined what the approximate length of each visit will be, this scheduling system can operate very efficiently.

Block Scheduling

The practitioner who utilizes this method of patient scheduling has several patients come in at the same time. A practitioner, for example, may tell three patients to come in at 10:00 A.M. Although the three patients arrive at the same time they will be seen only one at a time. This method of scheduling has the disadvantage of taking patients on a first-come, first-served basis. Patients may be forced to wait long periods if they arrive late. The method is advantageous to the practitioner since it generally assures there will be a patient waiting to be seen whenever the therapist becomes available.

Unit Scheduling or Patient Grouping

Patients seen utilizing this scheduling system are those who are to receive the same type of treatment. An example of this scheduling method would be to set aside Tuesday and Thursday afternoons for patients requiring only hand rehabilitation. The practitioner can work uninterrupted and concentrate on a specific treatment regime.

Modified or Rolling Wave System

The modified or rolling wave system is basically a modification of the block scheduling system. This system provides for the arrival of several patients over the span of fifteen to thirty minutes. It works particularly well where there are varying times in patient treatment.

Each hour is considered a block that is subdivided into several treatment periods. Shorter appointments are set at either the beginning or end of the hour. This method will provide the practitioner with a mix of patient treatments throughout the business day.

THE WAVE SYSTEM

1 pm	1:10 pm	1:30 pm
Re-check	Intermediate	New Patient

3pm		3:30pm	3:45pm
New Patient		Re-check	Re-check

Figure XXI. Each hour is considered a block which can be divided into different time slots depending on the rehabilitation needed and time to be alloted. Large periods of time can be set aside either at the beginning, middle, or end of the hour.

REDUCING NO-SHOWS

No matter how well the attempt to properly schedule patients there will always be an individual who either does not show up for a scheduled appointment or is so late that to attempt treatment would confuse the remainder of the day's schedule. The easier it is for a patient to arrive at any given time and receive treatment, the greater the tendency for a patient to not show up at a prescheduled appointment time. Anytime a patient can receive treatment by arriving late, the less the incentive to keep an appointment time.

Patients who arrive on time should not be made to wait while those who are late receive their treatments. In general, you are well within reason to refuse to see a patient who is ten minutes late. To accept a patient for treatment beyond that period of time rewards the person for their tardiness and angers those patients who arrive on time for their treatments.

When the receptionist schedules patients, have her inform them that the practice does run on time in providing patient treatments. Request the receptionist remind the patient at least twice of the specific time and date therapy is to be provided. To reduce repeated no-shows, some practitioners post signs which clearly indicate a fee will be charged for any appointment missed in which the practice did not receive advanced notification.

Patients who continually arrive late or do not show for appointments are often repeaters who represent only a small percentage of the patients seen by the practice. If the situation cannot be corrected, the practitioner should make sure there is sufficient documentation and then refuse to provide further treatments. The practitioner's final position should be communicated to the patient in writing. Depending on the situation, problem patients can also be informed that they must wait to be seen at the therapist's convenience. Long waiting periods can discourage tardiness.

HAVE PATIENTS FILL OUT
AN INFORMATION SHEET

It is essential that the practice is provided with information about the patient to be treated. Having each patient fill out an information sheet prior to offering treatment will tell you something about the individual and their personality.

ANYTOWN PHYSICAL THERAPY

PLEASE PRINT   PATIENT INFORMATION SHEET

Date: _____

Patient's Name _____
                    Last   First   Middle

Address _____
              Street   City   State   Zip Code

Telephone (Home) _____ (Work) _____

Age: _____ Birth Date: _____ Sex: _____ Status: M ___ S ___ W ___ D ___

Occupation: _____ Employer: _____

Employer's Address: _____
                         Street   City   State   Zip Code

Family Physician: _____ Referred By: _____

Parent's or Spouse's Name: _____ Phone: _____

Address: _____
              Street   City   State   Zip Code

Employer/Address: _____

Person Responsible for Payment: _____

Name & Address of Insurance Company: _____

_____

Policy #: _____ Social Security #: _____

Is this Workmen's Compensation? _____ Date of Accident: _____

Auto Accident? _____ Legal Action? _____

Allergies: _____

Present Complaint: _____

_____

Medicare Patients: I authorize any holder of medical or other information about me to release to the Social Security Administration and Health Care Financing Administration or its intermediaries or carriers any information needed for this or a related Medicare claim. I permit a copy of this authorization to be used in place of the original, and request payment of medical insurance benefits either to myself or to the party who accepts assignment.

Signature: _____ Date: _____

Other Insurance Companies: I authorize the release of any medical information necessary to process this claim and request payment of benefits either to myself or to the party who accepts assignment.

Signature: _____ Date: _____

I authorize payment of medical benefits directly to the physical therapist or medical facility for services described on health insurance claims form.

Signature: _____ Date: _____

If this is a workmen's compensation injury, please read and sign below:
Under penalty or perjury, I declare that the symptoms that I have related are, to the best of my knowledge and belief, due to a job related injury or illness.

Signature: _____ Date: _____

Figure XXII.

All patients should provide the practitioner with enough information to determine who will be paying for the physical therapy services to be provided. Many patients will automatically expect you to file their insurance for them but neglect to provide little if any information about the insurance company providing coverage.

The receptionist must check each patient information sheet to ascertain whether it is completely and properly filled out. Patients who refuse to provide essential information such as address, phone, place of employment, person responsible for payment, may also have no intention of paying their bill. When the necessary information cannot be obtained, offer to reschedule the patient for another appointment.

A PRACTICE INFORMATION BOOKLET

Many practitioners are providing patients with practice information booklets. The primary purpose of this material is to introduce a new patient to the practice and the services it has to offer. The booklet should be designed so as to save the patient and employees time in answering many of the questions which commonly arise. The booklet should also serve to improve patient/staff relations.

The material provided need not be detailed but instead, acquaint the new patient with the basic office policies and procedures. The booklet may be provided to each patient during their first visit or mailed to their home. Each booklet should provide a short introductory statement as indicated below.

PATIENT BOOKLET INTRODUCTORY LETTER

Welcome

Anytown Physical Therapy provides a highly trained staff to meet your rehabilitation needs. Family physicians and other medical specialists refer individuals to Anytown Physical Therapy for treatment of problems requiring specialized rehabilitation. After a complete evaluation, our physical therapists will work with you and your physician to provide the best care possible.

At Anytown Physical Therapy we know you have questions and concerns about your health care. We want you to have the answers to those questions and have prepared this booklet for your convenience. Of course, the staff will gladly help you with any questions not answered in the booklet.

THE BOOKLET SHOULD INCLUDE

1. Office phone numbers
2. Office hours
3. What information is needed to schedule appointments
4. How records are released
5. What the office policy is for payment of services
6. How fees are determined
7. What the office policy is on no-shows
8. A map which indicates practice location
9. What the best times are to call and speak with a therapist
10. What the policy is on providing information about the patient to others (employers, friends, etc.).

When printing a booklet, the practitioner should engage in comparison shopping. Look for a printer who does quality work at reasonable rates. Ask to see samples of similar work and have the costs of your printing needs estimated before agreeing to purchase. Often, for very little cost, a printer can reproduce your copy on colored paper or with colored ink.

If you plan a pamphlet for mass mailing, you can reduce the costs of envelopes by using a tri-folded sheet of paper. The paper should not be glued, stapled, or secured. In most instances this will be acceptable for regulation mailing. Consult your local post office for postage costs and regulations before printing.

CHAPTER EIGHT

HIRING PERSONNEL FOR THE PRACTICE

THE EMPLOYEES of a private practice are properly viewed as one of the most important assets. The success or failure of the practice will largely be determined by the caliber of the personnel hired and by the effort they exert. The selection of competent personnel need not be a difficult task. It is, however, essential you give careful consideration to each employee added to the practice. Poor judgement and haphazard selection techniques can create numerous problems in the office, antagonize patients, and contribute to a poor practice image. There are a number of methods to use in attracting and selecting competent office personnel. This chapter will provide general guidelines to the proper selection, evaluation, promotion, and dismissal of practice employees.

UNDERSTANDING WHAT IS NEEDED

The first step in successful staff selection is to decide what type of job you would like done and the characteristics of the individual needed to fill the job requirements. Without doing this, hiring frequently becomes haphazard with little analysis of the job to be filled and the training that will be required.

The primary objective of personnel selection is to attract and retain capable individuals. These individuals should be willing to work towards the promotion of practice growth while at the same time achieving practice objectives. The more the practitioner knows about the practice's projected growth and direction, the better the ability to judge what attributes will be required of employees.

Once you have an idea of the type of employee that will be needed, the next step is to specify in writing what will be the individual requirements. The requirements should include a list of the duties to be performed, the necessary educational requirements, and the experience needed.

Educational qualifications and work experience are important. The better the training and experience of the individual, the less the chance for error. There is, after all, very little room for error in a private practice.

Personality is also important because the employee will help set the atmosphere for the practice. An employee for a medical practice should be sincerely interested in people and willing to work toward practice objectives and goals. The employee will also serve a vital public relations role. They are often the first to greet the patient and convey the philosophy of the practice. How well they perform this function can win or lose patients.

REQUIREMENTS AND QUALIFICATIONS

Position: Physical Therapy Aide

Responsible To: Owner of Anytown Physical Therapy

Summary of Job: To assist the physical therapist and physical therapy assistant with patient treatment. Also responsible for the preparation and clean up of patient treatment rooms.

Specific Requirements:

1. Prepare, drape patients for treatment.
2. Assist in the transfer of patients.
3. Maintain inventory and supplies.
4. Perform clerical activities.

Job Qualifications: Prefer candidate with college course work in anatomy and physiology. Previous office experience also preferred. Accurate typing skills of not less than fifty words per minute required. Knowledge of medical office bookkeeping and business procedures also required.

Figure XXIII. Before interviewing any job candidate take a few moments to write down a brief job description. The description can later be expanded to include more duties and become part of the policies and procedures manual.

ATTRACTING THE RIGHT PERSON

Attracting the right person to the job begins with the advertisement of the job vacancy. Depending on the type of professional needed, many practitioners have found advertising in professional journals and magazines is the most effective. Nonprofessional personnel can be solicited through the local newspaper.

Development of a job advertisement requires as much effort as it does to determine the necessary qualifications. Proper wording of the advertisement will assist in the screening of applicants. For example, failure to indicate the location of the practice will result in a large number of responses from individuals who would not be interested in the job if it required them to relocate.

The advertisement should also state the hours of practice operation. If the practice is to be open on weekends, it should be specified. It is also important to indicate the type of patient most frequently treated by the practice. Indicating items such as these will help eliminate those applicants not genuinely interested in the practice opportunity.

Salary may be mentioned in professional advertisements, but it is not a requirement. The salary will always be negotiated depending upon the person to be hired. If your practice offers an excellent salary and benefit package do not hesitate to mention it in the advertisement. In the competitive health care industry, most employees expect good salaries and benefits.

THE INITIAL SCREENING OF APPLICANTS

A well written advertisement should attract a large number of interested applicants. Unless you want to spend a great deal of time personally discussing the job with each applicant, you should indicate in the advertisement to "Reply by telephone or resume." An initial screening of all applicants can be done quickly through the use of the telephone or resume.

The telephone can be an excellent means to screen a large number of candidates. A telephone conversation in a simple question and answer manner can detect obvious problems which would indicate someone is unsuitable for employment.

Use of a resume is a quick and relatively inexpensive means of obtaining valuable information about the applicant's ability to read and write. If the resume is sloppy, chances are the individual's work habits will be very similar. The resume will also give some idea of an applicant's previous work experience, education, and interests. This helps to provide the practitioner with a starting point for discussion should there be an interview.

WHEN USING RESUMES, CONDUCT A PRESCREENING INTERVIEW

After you have reviewed the resumes and selected the most qualified applicants, the next step is to contact each by telephone. The telephone call will allow you to evaluate the individual's voice and attitude as well as their availability for interview.

The prescreening interview is especially important if you plan to provide reimbursement for interview expenses. Interviewing takes considerable time away from the treatment of patients. Prescreening allows the list to be further narrowed so only those individuals most qualified will be interviewed.

THE EMPLOYMENT INTERVIEW

Once the list of applicants has been narrowed to those whom you want to personally interview, arrange a mutually convenient time. In most employment interview sessions, the practitioner should set aside approximately thirty minutes to no more than one hour. The interview should be conducted at the practice facility so that a tour of the working environment can also be provided.

The employment interview is important since it will provide a face-to-face encounter for evaluation of the perspective candidate's personality. The conversation should be directed by the practitioner, but give the applicant sufficient time to talk during the interview. The more the individual is allowed to talk, the more that can be determined about the candidate's communication skills and demeanor.

Question the applicant about what they liked or disliked about a previous position. One mistake frequently encountered is the asking of questions which suggest the correct answer. For example, asking a physical therapist if he/she likes working with amputee patients will likely obtain a "yes" response if the person really wants the job. However, if you were to ask the individual to list their most favorite and least favorite type of patient, it may provide another response.

Attempt to conduct the interview at a time when the office will be quiet. The best times are usually early in the morning or after the completion of office hours. It costs money to hire an employee so it is essential you provide a relaxed atmosphere in which to judge the applicants overall ability. Do not be in a hurry to hire an employee. Selection of the wrong personnel can result in a continuous process of interviewing and selecting employees. This adds to practice expenses.

Before each applicant arrives for interview, review the job description and their resume. If there are gaps where there was no period of employment this should be questioned. You may wish to provide the applicant with a copy of the job description to stimulate questions about the job and its requirements.

Throughout the interview, emphasize eye contact and a sincere willingness to listen. If possible, try not to sit behind a desk during the question and answer periods. This typically will hinder the free exchange of information.

CHECK THE REFERENCES

An investigation into a promising candidate's background is too often overlooked by the private practitioner. No matter how well the applicant does in the interview, make every effort to check the references provided. The best guide to what an employee will do in the future is by what has been done in the past. Asking the proper questions of former employers requires little time or money, but is worth the effort.

There are four categories for obtaining background information on a perspective candidate. They are:

1. School officials
2. Former employers
3. Character references
4. Neighbors of the applicant

The third category is generally unreliable. Very few perspective employees will list an individual on a resume who will provide anything other than an excellent reference. For this reason, character references can generally be eliminated.

The fourth category "neighbors," may also be very unreliable. Most of these individuals know the applicant as a "nice guy," but have never been in a position to evaluate the person's work or their employment history.

If the person has recently graduated from high school or college, it is advisable to contact those individuals who provided instruction. Information can be obtained relative to attendance, grade point average, level of aspiration, motivation, and emotional adjustment.

Former employers are the most valuable. They are in a position to provide information regarding the quantity and quality of work produced, dependability, initiative, and the relationships with fellow employees and supervisors.

It is advisable to call the references listed rather than mail a questionnaire. Previous employers are sometimes reluctant to write down information which is negative. Many will, however, be quite honest over the telephone.

When contacting a perspective candidate's former employer, prepare a brief list of questions which will require only a yes or no response. Do not ask a former employer to elaborate on any one question. If they hesitate or refuse to answer a question, try to remember to listen for "What is not said but what is implied." Do not, however, let one disgruntled former employer ruin the chances for employment of a good applicant. Develop a list of phone questions such as shown in Figure XXIV.

PREVIOUS EMPLOYER REFERENCE LIST

Date Called _____

Name _____ Position _____

Previous Employer _____ Person Interviewed _____

Job Title _____

QUESTIONS   REMARKS

1. How long did the applicant work for you?

2. Was the employee reliable, loyal and diligent?

3. Was the employee good with patients?

4. Did the employee handle stressful situations well?

5. Was the employee honest?

6. Did the employee get along with fellow staff members?

7. Did the employee display leadership qualities?

8. Could the employee follow instructions?

9. Would you say the employee's work was above average, average, or below average?

10. Would you rehire the employee?

Figure XXIV. The answers provided will provide a general guideline to an applicant's past employment performance. Before contacting the current or former employer obtain written approval from the applicant.

A SECOND INTERVIEW

When the field of possible applicants has been narrowed to the final few, contact each potential employee for a second interview. The second interview will allow you to ask questions not covered during the first session.

A perspective employee, under serious consideration, should be seen at least twice. The second interview will make certain the applicant comes across the same way both times. The final interview should also fully explain the practice working hours, employee benefits and salary, as well as any job requirements which may need further clarification.

REJECTING UNQUALIFIED APPLICANTS

One of the most difficult tasks for many practitioners is to notify an applicant that he or she will not be hired by the practice. To notify the applicant is only common courtesy. There is a tendency to reject the applicant very lightly with statements such as, "We really liked you and hope to be hiring additional personnel soon." If, however, you are sure you will not be hiring soon, do not allow this person to hold out hope that you will be calling.

It is essential to maintain the goodwill of the practice when rejecting an applicant. The rejection should not reflect poorly on the practice nor damage the self-concept of the individuals being rejected. There are a number of ways to inform an applicant that the practice will not be hiring them.

If the applicant can clearly see that his or her interests or salary needs are incompatible with the situation, the individual may reject himself/herself by gracefully withdrawing. If the individual possesses the necessary qualifications but does not match the particular job, they should be informed that their particular skills and abilities are good, but that they do not match what the practice requires.

When the person possesses all the required skills and abilities but the personality of the individual does not meet the practice requirements, this presents a more difficult problem. Since mere personality cannot be objectively measured, there is a potential to create the feeling of discrimination if denied a job solely for this reason. The situation requires skill on the part of the practitioner to carefully convey the reason why the applicant is being rejected. In situations such as these it may be best to imply that the search is going to continue for sometime until all avenues have been investigated.

HAVE A PROBATIONARY PERIOD

Every new employee should be given a probationary period before final acceptance as a staff member. The period may be a few weeks or as much as ninety days. During the probationary period, the practitioner should closely monitor individual performance.

The employee should be advised from the very beginning of employment that there is a trial period. If at any time throughout this period the practitioner is not satisfied with the new employee's performance, the individual should be informed. Poor performance should be given the opportunity to be rectified. If the warning does not correct the problem then the employee should be terminated.

Once the probationary period has ended, you should review the job performance of the individual and express your satisfaction. Some practitioners use a standardized performance appraisal. Others develop one to meet their practice needs. In either case, provide a blank copy to the employee at the time of employment in order to show them how they will be evaluated.

TRAINING THE EMPLOYEE

Too often a new employee is hired without a complete understanding of the job to be performed. Many times, the new person is hired and everyone in the office assumes the person will learn as they go along. This frequently makes the new employee very uncomfortable and often somewhat resentful of being provided with little or no direction.

Training a new employee requires the practitioner to be both understanding and patient. There are a number of ways to provide a new employee with job training. One method is to assign the new staff member to another employee who is very familiar with practice operations. This will allow the new employee to ask questions as they go about learning their job responsibilities. The assignment of the new staff member to the established staff member should only be done if it is reasonably certain the two employees will interact well together.

Another method is for the practitioner, or the person who hired the new employee, to assume the sole responsibility for the training program. This method has the advantage of allowing the practitioner to show, rather than describe, the operations of the practice. This method can also help the new employee gain confidence as long as praise is liberal and positive.

A new job is stressful for an employee. Always try to stress the importance of detail in patient treatment. An employee should be corrected when a mistake is made but not in front of patients or fellow employees. If the employee is well trained, he or she will quickly become an important asset to the practice. The practitioner who properly and thoroughly develops the employees will increase their confidence level. Proper training allows each member of the practice to know what is expected and what constitutes high quality patient care.

THE PERFORMANCE APPRAISAL

Practitioners who evaluate the staff on a regular basis help create an office atmosphere in which the employees feel their efforts are noticed and appreciated. The failure to demonstrate gratitude for an employee's actions can lead to employee dissatisfaction and job disillusionment. The lack of feedback about job performance can greatly lower the morale of the entire office.

Performance evaluations and salary reviews should be done on a regular basis. It is, however, recommended to separate the performance evaluation from the salary review. If not, the employee frequently anticipates the news of the increase in salary rather than concentrating on how the job could be done better. Listed below are some general guidelines to follow in the performance evaluation.

1. Ask the employee how the job is going. What areas of the job need to be improved? Can you provide any recommendations as to how these can be changed?
2. Ask the employee to comment on each area of evaluation.
3. Stress the things the employee does well.
4. When discussing employee weaknesses, encourage the employee to offer suggestions for change.
5. Set a date to reevaluate the changes that are to be made.
6. Try to end the evaluation on a positive note. If possible, express appreciation for the job the employee is doing.

As described in Figure XXV, the type of performance appraisal can vary. The performance appraisal used for the evaluation of a new employee can also be used to evaluate an established employee. Regardless of the type of appraisal form implemented, the goal of the appraisal is to aid in creating and maintaining a satisfactory level of performance by all practice employees.

SAMPLE PERFORMANCE APPRAISAL

Name _____

Position _____

Date of Evaluation _____

Job Knowledge

1	2	3	4	5
Serious gaps in his knowledge of essentials of job	Satisfactory knowledge of routine aspects of job	Adequately informed on most phases of job	Good knowledge of all phases of job	Excellent understanding of his job. Extremely well informed

Judgment

1	2	3	4	5
Decisions often wrong or ineffective	Judgment often sound but makes some errors	Good decisions resulting from sound analysis of factors	Sound, logical thinker	Consistently makes sound decisions, even on complex issues

Oral and Written Communication

1	2	3	4	5
Unable to express ideas clearly. Often misunderstood	Expresses ideas satisfactorily on routine topics	Generally expresses thoughts adequately	Consistently expresses thoughts clearly	Outstanding in written and oral expression

Attitude

1	2	3	4	5
Uncooperative, resents suggestions, no enthusiasm	Often cooperates, often accepts suggestions	Satisfactory cooperation, accepts new ideas	Responsive, cooperates well, helpful to others	Excellent in cooperation, welcomes new ideas, very helpful and enthusiastic

Quantity of Work

1	2	3	4	5
Fails below minimum requirements	Usually meets minimum requirements	Satisfactory quantity	Usually well exceeds minimum	Consistently produces superior quantity

Quality of Work

1	2	3	4	5
Poor quality, many errors or rejects	Quality usually o.k. Some errors or rejects	Satisfactory quality	Quality exceeds normal standards	Consistent high quality work

Overall Evaluation

1	2	3	4	5
Poor	Fair	Satisfactory	Good	Excellent

Comments _____

_____

_____

Employee Signature _____

Employer Signature _____

Figure XXV. There are many types of performance appraisals. The conventional rating scale uses five categories for each factor being rated.

PROMOTING STAFF MEMBERS

The selection of employees for promotion is very closely related to the performance appraisal. You want to promote those individuals who exhibit the traits, characteristics, and skills necessary to undertake added job responsibilities.

Some practitioners automatically consider the employee who has been there the longest as the best candidate for promotion. The basis of the selection is therefore based on seniority. The person selected, however, may have no interest in taking on additional responsibilities.

Seniority has several possible side effects. One side effect is that it may result in the selection of an unqualified person occupying an important position. The seniority method can also lead to morale problems and a loss in practice efficiency. An employee may loose the incentive to excel if it is well known that excellence does not count towards promotion. Ambitious employees will get discouraged and may potentially leave the practice if they know they must wait years before being promoted.

When considering the promotion of one of the members of the practice let all members of the practice know in advance. This will allow volunteers to come forward and offer to take the position. This helps to ascertain which members are interested and which are not. Following this recommendation helps to prevent the sometimes embarrassing situation where you ask an employee who subsequently turns down your promotion opportunity.

To properly assess any candidate for promotion there are three areas of employee qualifications which must be evaluated. These are the individual's technical abilities, ability to supervise others, and the individual's personality traits.

Technical Competence

For any supervisory position there must be an ability to analyze individual job requirements and act in a manner which helps to promote the accomplishment of practice objectives and goals. To be considered for promotion, an employee should demonstrate excellence in the performance of a job and have a proven record of assuming greater responsibility.

Ability to Supervise Others

Supervision is the process of leading, coordinating, and directing the work of the practice employees. An individual in a supervisory position guides fellow employees so they produce the desired quality of health care. The individual under consideration for promotion must be the type that understands fellow employees have lives outside the office environment. The same person must also recognize, and if necessary deal with, those individuals who take advantage of their employment opportunity. The candidate will be required to guide employees in the scheduling of work, set a consistent example of proper performance, and above all demonstrate a willingness to listen to employee suggestions.

Personality Traits

The candidate must demonstrate loyalty to the office. Good supervision is often complicated and frequently requires an individual who will strive to keep the practice owner satisfied as well as the fellow employees and patients.

Communication skills are essential. The person chosen for promotion will speak on behalf of the practice to the public and the employees. The candidate's attitude towards their job will often be demonstrated by their communication skills and ability to interact with others. Taking time to listen to the office conversations will be helpful in judging communication skills.

HOW AND WHEN TO TERMINATE A STAFF MEMBER

One of the most difficult managerial functions for the private practitioner is to release an employee from employment. When the situation reaches the point where an employee must be let go there is often a very uncomfortable feeling throughout the entire office.

There are a number of reasons why an employee can and should be terminated. Some, such as embezzlement, require immediate action. Others, such as a poor attitude, may need only to be corrected. There are no simple solutions. Each requires careful analysis of the problem before taking any action.

THE PROBATIONARY PERIOD

When an employee is new and simply lacks the necessary skills for the job you have one of two alternatives. You can work with the individual to correct the deficiency or dismiss them from employment. Lack of ability can, however, be confused with inexperience. If the employee is having only small problems with adjustment it may be advisable to work out the problems rather than go through the expensive and time consuming process of locating another employee.

The best time to release any undesirable employee is during the probationary period. Every new employee should have a thorough understanding that the first few weeks or months of employment will be probationary. The probationary period allows you to closely monitor the performance of the employee before making them a permanent staff member. If it is apparent that the new employee will not be acceptable, they should not be kept on staff.

TERMINATION OF THE ESTABLISHED EMPLOYEE

In situations where the employee has been with the practice for several years, the dismissal process is often more difficult. When presented with this situation, you must express your dissatisfaction and provide the employee with enough time to correct the problem. Employees often have problems outside of work which can affect job performance. In many instances, just letting the employee know that you are unhappy with their performance will correct the problem behavior.

When the problem is not easily corrected, the employee should first be warned that the behavior is not appropriate. This discussion should be noted in the employee's file, including the date the warning was given, what transpired in the conversation, and what solutions were posed.

If the problem continues, a written warning should be given to the employee. The warning should once again describe the behavior which needs to be changed. A time frame for correction of the behavior should also be indicated. The written warning should be signed and dated by the employee. Once again, all warnings should become a part of the employee's permanent file.

When an employee receives a written warning most will take corrective action immediately. When they do not, the next step is termination. The termination of an employee may or may not follow the three-step procedure described. The employment situation may indicate that more warnings should be given. No matter how many warnings are given, documentation is essential in the event the employee accuses the practitioner of unfair labor practices.

THE TERMINATION INTERVIEW

Once the decision is made to terminate an employee the next step is to determine an appropriate time and place to inform the individual. In terminating any employee the practitioner must first consider the impact the action will have on the practice. To do this, the practitioner must decide whether the employee should be dismissed now, at the end of the week, or when an appropriate replacement is found. The impact of the termination may be difficult on the rest of the staff, since they will be required to perform the functions of the terminated employee.

In terminating an employee, always attempt to conduct a termination interview. The interview provides the employee with the specific reasons for dismissal. All termination interviews should be conducted in a quiet place away from staff members and patients. It can be conducted very professionally by following a few simple steps.

1. **Be Direct.** Tell the employee that, despite the effort on both sides, the job has not been to your satisfaction.

2. **Indicate the Finality of the Decision.** Any pleas for another chance should be disregarded. You have already done everything you can.

3. **Remain Brief.** Meetings such as these should remain brief. Repeated discussions of weaknesses, already identified, may lead to employee anger and hostility.

4. **Emphasize Good Points.** Soothing an ego can be beneficial. Reinforce the positive areas of the employee's work that can be taken to the next job.

5. **Tell the Employee When the Termination Is Effective.** In most instances the termination will be immediately effective. Unless there is a specific duty which must be completed, the employee should leave at the end of the interview.

6. **Give Some Idea of the Type of Reference You Will Provide.** Tell the person exactly what reason will be given for dismissal.

7. **Discuss the Severance Package.** The severance package can include a number of monetary items. In most cases, the employee should be provided with one to two weeks salary depending on the length of notice.

8. **Discuss Who Should Inform the Staff.** This can be avoided if the dismissal is done at the end of the day. However, do not terminate an employee without having someone else present as a witness.

9. **Express Your Best Wishes in Future Employment Opportunities.**

10. **Document as Much of the Conversation as Possible.** Include all comments made by both parties.

THE DISMISSAL PACKAGE

Before terminating the employee the practitioner should prepare the severance package. The severance package includes all monies owed to the employee. These include such items as salary, vacation, unused sick leave, and money in lieu of notice.

THE DISMISSAL PACKAGE

Employee _____ Date _____

The following items were discussed with the employee and met with his or her satisfaction.

Salary (year to date)   _____
Hourly Rate   _____

Accrued Vacation $_____Per Hr. X ___Days   _____
Accrued Sick Leave $_____Per Hr. X ___Days   _____
Severance Pay $_____Per Hr. X ___Days   _____

                              TOTAL $_____

Employee paid by check number _____

Keys issued at employment   _____
Keys returned at dismissal   _____

Employee Signature _____ Date _____

Supervisor Signature _____ Date _____

Witness Signature _____ Date _____

Figure XXVI. One copy should be given to the employee. A second copy should be maintained in the employee's permanent file.

You should be prepared to discuss how the group health and life insurance offered by the practice can be converted to an individual policy if the employee is interested. In a situation where the employee is vested in a profit-sharing or pension program, it should be discussed with the practice accountant before meeting with the employee.

The termination package should be carefully spelled out in writing and signed by the employee. This prevents problems should compensation questions arise in the future. Prior to requesting the employee's signature, ask for any keys belonging to the practice.

THE POSSIBLE PROBLEMS WITH DISMISSAL

Even though it may not be apparent at the exit interview, some employees may become very angry after being terminated. There are a number of ways a former employee can strike back at the practice. It is important to be aware of the problems which can be created, and how to handle them once they occur.

After dismissal, the employee may file for unemployment compensation. Depending on the reason for dismissal the employee may not be entitled to benefits. If the employee was dismissed for improper conduct, made false statements in order to collect benefits, or quit for no apparent reason, they generally are not entitled to benefits. Once the dismissed employee is offered suitable work by the state employment agency they must accept the position or risk loss of benefits. It is advisable, however, not to attempt to force an employee to quit to avoid paying unemployment.

When an employee feels the job loss was due to discrimination there could be a lawsuit. Proper documentation for the specific reason of dismissal becomes important if age, sex, religion, race, or national origin can be implied as factors which influenced the termination decision.

Once discharged, an employee can claim there was sexual harassment. One of the greatest mistakes an employer can make is to become emotionally involved with a staff member. Practice relationships should be friendly but never romantic. If you have never shown any signs of emotional involvement with an employee, the remaining staff should be able to attest to your innocence.

Disgruntled employees can also file a claim with workers' compensation stating they were released due to injury. This can be avoided by making sure each injury, no matter how seemingly insignificant, is documented in the employee's file. In no instances should an employee be terminated due to injury. Instead, hire a temporary replacement and put the injured worker on inactive status. In some states it is illegal to dismiss any employee due to injury no matter how much work is missed. Workers' compensation will eventually determine if the employee will be returning to work.

A former employee can also begin to spread rumors about you and the practice. Unless you can prove the rumors are costing you patients and income it is best to do nothing. Most individuals will recognize the derogatory statements as coming from a disgruntled former employee. Few will give them any serious credence.

KEEPING THE STAFF SATISFIED

There are many sources of satisfaction that can be derived from working in a private practice. The physical therapist who can compliment the staff and provide opportunities for professional growth and development will contribute to increasing employee morale and satisfaction.

One of the best ways to keep a good staff is to conduct performance and salary reviews on a regular basis. Always try to reinforce good performance and encourage better performance. A raise in salary, a periodic bonus, an extra afternoon off, all tell employees that you recognize their efforts and that you care.

Making a sincere effort to demonstrate a caring attitude will be reflected in the quality of care delivered to the patient. The patients will, in turn, express their appreciation through repeated office visits. The secret to building a loyal, devoted, and hardworking office team begins with the sincere effort of the practice owner.

CHAPTER NINE

PRIVATE PRACTICE BOOKKEEPING, PATIENT BILLING, AND COLLECTIONS

THE PHYSICAL therapist as owner of a small business must be in a position to evaluate the financial situation of the practice at any time. There is a close relationship between sound practice bookkeeping principles and profitability. In fact, evidence indicates that poor financial bookkeeping may lead to business failure. It is therefore important that a private practitioner establish a comprehensive and useful bookkeeping system that is understandable and easy to interpret.

A steady stream of income allows the practice to continue operations. A good bookkeeping system requires careful planning to establish a proper routine for handling all money collected by the practice. This chapter discusses the acceptable methods for bookkeeping, patient billing, the use of a collection agency, and methods to use in determining and preventing employee embezzlement. Proper bookkeeping is essential to effective financial decision making. A practitioner who bases financial decisions upon inadequate and unreliable bookkeeping information is inviting trouble.

THE BASIC BOOKKEEPING RECORDS

A well designed system of bookkeeping provides three objectives to a physical therapy practice. The first objective is to provide a record of all financial transactions so as to allow the practitioner to prepare financial statements and reports. For tax purposes it is essential there be a record for every business transaction.

The second objective of a bookkeeping system is for business planning. Accurate financial records are an indispensable tool for telling the practitioner where the practice is going. Each practitioner should know how much has been collected, how much is outstanding, and how much is owed. Without a good system of financial bookkeeping the practitioner is unable to assess the financial progress of the practice.

The third objective of proper bookkeeping methods is to protect the practice assets from being misstated through carelessness, errors, and fraud. The practitioner invests considerable time and effort in practice operations in hopes of returning a reasonable profit. Complete and accurate records will act as a protective device against the inefficient use of resources, fraud, theft, and waste by practice employees.

Every physical therapy practice should include the following financial records:

1. **Day Sheet (Daily Business Summary).** The day sheet provides a detailed daily listing of all patients seen, the amount they were charged for services, and the amount of money that was collected. The day sheet should be totaled at the end of each business day. Each sheet should provide information about how much money was collected by cash and check as well as how much is still owed. Day sheets may be obtained from any small business supply store. (See Figure XXVII.)

2. **Patient Charge Tickets.** The charge ticket is a itemized statement of the services the patient received and their cost. The ticket will provide a method of communication between the practitioner and the staff member who is responsible for practice bookkeeping and patient billing. (See Figure XXVIII.)

3. **Ledger Cards.** The ledger card represents an individual account receivable. Each card is a record of the services provided to a patient showing the fees for services, how much has been paid, and how much is still owed. The ledger card can be photocopied and mailed to a patient when requesting payment for services. (See Figure XXIX.)

4. **Disbursement Journal.** A disbursement journal provides a detailed listing of all outgoing cash and checks. The journal may be maintained in conjunction with the practice checkbook. (See Figure XXX.)

5. **Payroll Ledger.** The payroll ledger is a record of each employee's wages and withholdings. Maintaining a payroll ledger will provide a convenient basis for the preparation of federal, state, and local tax reports. The practitioner can also maintain a record of hours worked and overtime earnings. (See Figure XXXI.)

DAY SHEET (Daily Business Summary) — EXAMPLE

SHEET NO. _____ OF _____   DATE: 9/5/XX

DATE	DESCRIPTION	CHARGE	CREDITS Payment	CREDITS Adj.	CURRENT BALANCE	PREVIOUS BALANCE	NAME	RECEIPT NUMBER	CASH	CHECKS	BUSINESS ANALYSIS SUMMARIES (OPTIONAL)
9/5	Ther Ex	25.00	25.00		-0-	-0-	O.R. Johnson	0915		25.00	
9/5	HP/US/Ex	45.00	20.00		25.00	-0-	B.P. Jones	0916	25.00		
9/5	HP/US/CT	45.00	25.00		20.00	-0-	H.I. Gentry	0917		20.00	
9/5	US/Ther Ex	35.00	20.00		50.00	35.00	J. Dickens	0918	20.00		
9/5	Ther Ex	25.00	25.00		-0-	-0-	G. Gentle	0919		25.00	
9/5	Ther Ex	25.00	25.00		25.00	25.00	H.C. Smith	0920		25.00	
9/5	Ther Ex	25.00	25.00		-0-	-0-	C. Sykes	0921	25.00		
9/5	US/Ther Ex	35.00	25.00		10.00	-0-	M. Green	0922	25.00		
9/5	Eval	35.00			85.00	50.00	N. Poole	0923			
9/5	Ins Payment		85.00		15.00	100.00	I. Hinkle	0924		85.00	
9/5	Ins Payment		50.00		-0-	50.00	G. Swanson	0925		50.00	
9/5	Ins Payment		20.00		-0-	20.00	W. Willis	0926		20.00	
9/5	Ins Payment		100.00		50.00	150.00	J. Doe	0927		100.00	

	Col A	Col B-1	Col B-2	Col C	Col D
TOTALS THIS PAGE	295.00	445.00	-0-	280.00	430.00
PREVIOUS PAGE	2000.00	1500.00	125.00	615.00	240.00
MONTH-TO-DATE	2295.00	1945.00	125.00	895.00	670.00

	CASH	CHECKS
TOTALS	95.00	350.00

TOTAL DEPOSIT $ 445.00

PROOF OF POSTING

COL. D TOTAL	$ 430.00
PLUS COL. A TOTAL	$ 295.00
SUB TOTAL	$ 725.00
LESS COLS. B-1 & B-2	$ 445.00
MUST EQUAL COL. C	$ 280.00

ACCOUNTS RECEIVABLE CONTROL

PREVIOUS DAY'S TOTAL	$ 3375.00
PLUS COL A	$ 295.00
SUB TOTAL	$ 3670.00
LESS COLS. B-1 & B-2	$ 445.00
TOTAL ACCTS. REC.	$ 3225.00

ACCOUNTS RECEIVABLE PROOF

ACCTS. REC. 1ST OF MONTH	$ 3000.00
PLUS COL. A - MO. TO DATE	$ 2295.00
SUB TOTAL	$ 5295.00
LESS B-1 & B-2 MO. TO DATE	$ 2070.00
TOTAL ACCTS. REC.	$ 3225.00

CASH PAID OUT

Postage	$ 10.00
	$ 10.00

CASH CONTROL

Beginning Cash On Hand	$ 50.00
Receipts Today (Col. "B-1")	$ 445.00
Total	$ 495.00
Less Paid Out	$ 10.00
Less Bank Deposit	$ 445.00
Closing Cash On Hand	$ 40.00

Figure XXVII.

DATE	FAMILY MEMBER	DESCRIPTION	CHARGE	PAYMENT	ADJ CREDITS	CURRENT BALANCE	PREVIOUS BALANCE	NAME

This is your RECEIPT for this amount ▲

▲ This is a STATEMENT of your account to date

THERAPEUTIC EXERCISE
( ) 97110 Supervised
( ) 97145 Each Additional 15 Min.
HYDROTHERAPY
( ) 97022 Whirlpool
( ) 97022 Whirlpool – Sterile
( )
TRACTION
( ) 97012 Traction – Mechanical
( ) 97122 Traction – Manual
PHYSICAL MEDICINE
( ) 97124 Massage, One body part
( ) 97139 Unlisted Procedure (Specify)
( ) 97010 Hot Packs

( ) 97010 Cold Packs
( ) 97128 Ultrasound
( ) 97118 Electrical Stimulation
( )
( ) 97145 Treatment to one area
( ) Each additional 15 min.
( ) 97116 Gait Training
( )
( )
( ) 97039 Unlisted modality (specify)
KINETIC EXERCISE
( )
( ) 97740 Kinetic Exercise (30 Min.)
( ) 97741 Kinetic Exercise (Add'l 15 min)
( )

MISCELLANEOUS
( ) 97700 Evaluation
( ) 97540 ADL
( ) 90120 Home Visit
( ) 06506 Delivery charge for equip.
( ) E1399 CPM Rental
( )
( ) 90260 Hospital Visits
( )
( )
( )

PLACE OF SERVICE: ( ) Office   ( ) Hospital   ( ) Home   ( ) Other

DIAGNOSIS: _____

Anytown Physical Therapy Clinic
Anytown, USA

NEXT APPOINTMENT _____   AT _____   A.M. P.M.

Figure XXVIII.

STATEMENT
Anytown Physical Therapy Clinic

Brian Brown
247 Holiday Park Blvd.
Anytown, USA XX000

19XX

BAL. FWD. →

DATE	FAMILY MEMBER	DESCRIPTION	CHARGE	CREDITS		CURRENT BALANCE
				PAYMENTS	ADJ.	
6/18		WP²⁰ EX²⁵	45 00			45 00
6/20		EX	25 00			70 00
6/21		EX	25 00			95 00
6/24		EX	25 00			120 00
6/25		EX	25 00			145 00
7/1		Statement Sent				
7/5		Pt. Check		145 00		—0—

PLEASE PAY THE LAST FIGURE IN THIS COLUMN ▲

THIS IS A PHOTO COPY OF YOUR ACCOUNT AS IT APPEARS ON YOUR LEDGER CARD

Figure XXIX.

DISBURSEMENT JOURNAL

Date 19	Payee	Check Number	Post	Check Amount (Cr.)	Accounts Payable (Dr.)	Gross Pay (Dr.)	Social Security	Federal Income Taxes	State Income Taxes	Hosp.	Other Operating Expenses (Dr.)	Account	Amount
								Wages and Salaries — Deductions (Cr.)				**Other Disbursements**	
8/1	NASH SUPPLIES	2056		2500	3000							CASH DIS.	500.00
8/3	SUE BROWN	2057		128.85		24000	17.40	60.00	3.75	30.00			
8/3	BOB JONES	2058		59.62		9000	6.53	22.50	1.35	-0-			
	POSTAGE	2079		10.00							10.00		
	MONTHLY TOTALS			14829.62	8260.85	140000	101.50	35000	21.00	120.00	4260.28		520.00

Figure XXX.

PAYROLL LEDGER

Name **Sue Brown**

Address **12 E. 10th. St.**

West End, Tenn

Soc. Sec. No. **999-99-999**

Date of Birth **4-8-42**

No. of Exemptions **0 (Single)**   Wage Rate **6.00/hr.**

Pay Period Ending	\ Hours Worked \ S	M	T	W	Th	F	S	Total Reg. Hours	Earnings Overtime	Regular Rate	Overtime Rate	Total	Deductions Social Security	Fed. Income Tax	State Income Tax	Other	Net Pay
8/31-		8	8	8	8	8		40		240.00		240.00	17.40	60.00	3.75	30.00	128.85
8/10-		4	8	8	8	8		36		216.00		216.00	15.66	54.00	3.24	30.00	113.10
QUARTERLY TOTALS												3055.00	221.49	763.75	45.83	39.00	1633.93

Figure XXXI.

Good bookkeeping practices are essential in any successful practice. The expense associated with employing an experienced accountant for initial bookkeeping purposes will be a worthwhile investment. Accountants can provide a wide range of services including the actual setup of the books for a new practice.

Having an accountant provide all the bookkeeping services can be expensive. To reduce costs, the practitioner may consider keeping most of the daily records and then periodically turning them over to the accountant for in-depth analysis. The accountant can then prepare financial statements and tax reports for much less than it would cost to provide a complete accounting service.

MAINTAINING PETTY CASH AND PROVIDING CHANGE

In all small business situations there will be instances when a staff member must purchase supplies for the practice or provide change to a patient who is making a cash payment. To do this the practice must maintain small amounts of cash on a daily basis.

Maintaining a petty cash fund in the office will allow staff members to purchase small items without the necessity of obtaining a check from the practitioner. For most practice situations fifty to seventy-five dollars is sufficient to allow for small purchases. Each time a purchase is made a receipt should be obtained and the amount recorded in a petty cash booklet. The information recorded in the booklet should include the date, item, and the name of the person making the purchase.

To adequately make change, the practitioner should maintain fifty to seventy-five dollars in small bills. The money from the accounts must never be combined. Money from both accounts should be kept in a locked desk drawer or office safe.

PATIENT BILLING AND COLLECTIONS

Collecting for services requires a special effort by all staff members. Ask staff members what they like least about working in a private practice and most will say, "patient billing and collections." Because of this, personnel often give this important task low priority. It is often a difficult task to put pressure on patients. Consequently, whenever possible the task is ignored.

The success of any collection system is measured by the collection percentage. The practitioner can easily determine whether collection efforts are successful by using a simple mathematical formula. The formula is as follows:

$$\frac{\text{Amount Collected}}{\text{Amount Billed}} \times 100 = \text{Collection Percentage}$$

The collection percentage will vary depending on the type of patient treatment and the fee charged. Insurance companies may adjust fees downward, such as workers' compensation, if they are considered excessive. Most practitioners should attempt to collect at least 90 percent. First year practitioners will have lower collection percentages since there are more charges at the end of the year than at the beginning. The percentage is lower because there has not been enough time to collect for all services.

Collecting for services is vital to achieving a successful business operation. In most cases, the success of a practice's billing and collection efforts will be contingent upon staff efforts in three important areas. They are:

1. **Always attempt to explain to the patient what services they will be paying for.** The best time to explain costs is when a new patient asks for an appointment. Each patient is entitled to know what services they will be receiving and how much is their estimated cost. The patient who knows in advance how much a service will be is less likely to refuse to make a payment.

2. **Itemize all treatments when provided.** Few insurance companies will accept billings which are lumped together. The charge ticket provides a simple means of itemizing all patient services. Complete with insurance codes, the ticket makes it much easier for the patient to be reimbursed for physical therapy services provided.

3. **Send all billing statements on a regular basis.** Do not allow an account to become long over-due before attempting to contact the patient. The regular billing of patients helps discourage them from falling behind in their payment schedule. The practitioner who bills on an irregular basis can expect the patients to respond in a similar manner. The longer the time lapse between billings the less likely the account will be paid.

Encourage each patient to make a payment on a specific date. When sending bills through the mail always enclose a self-addressed envelope. The envelope helps to further emphasize that payment is expected.

SETTING UP THE COLLECTION PROCEDURE

When each patient has completed a treatment session they should be presented with an itemized statement, signed by the therapist, which indicates the treatment received. This statement should be taken to the receptionist so appropriate fees can be determined.

In most instances the patient will be prepared to make a payment. When the patient does pay they should be presented with a receipted charge ticket as a record of payment. The receipt the patient receives will be forwarded by the patient to their insurance company.

In some cases, however, the patient will not be prepared to pay. In either instance, when the patient arrives at the receptionist's desk it is her responsibility to make the first move. A statement such as, "The fee for today's physical therapy services is twenty-five dollars" is all that should be said. Based on this statement, the patient should be willing to make a payment.

When not prepared to make a payment, the patient will often respond, "I didn't bring any money with me" or "Could you just send me a bill?" When either of these statements are made it is important that the receptionist emphasize that payment, even if only partial payment, is expected at the time of service. The receptionist should then respond by handing the patient a self-addressed envelope and asking them to mail payment as soon as they return home.

When a patient responds to the request for payment such as, "Can you file my insurance?", once again have the receptionist remind the patient that you expect payment at the time of service. The receptionist should respond with willingness to complete the form and assist in any way possible, but the patient should understand it is not the policy of the office to process insurance paperwork as the only means to obtain payment.

WHEN PAYMENT IS NOT RECEIVED

When billing statements have been sent to patients and no replies have been received the practitioner must then begin more aggressive tactics to collect for services. Patients may refuse to pay for physical therapy for a number of reasons. The most common are: (1) irresponsible, (2) financially unable, (3) never plan to pay.

In situations where the patient is irresponsible, it may be that they are putting off payment in order to pay other bills. Patients such as these will respond well to regular billing and collection efforts. Many of these individuals will finally make all their payments but will often need continued encouragement in order to do so.

Patients who are financially unable to pay may earnestly want to make payments but have run into difficulties. In situations such as these the patient will frequently respond by requesting to make payments on an installment basis. Depending on how the situation is handled the practitioner who agrees to accept installment payments may come under the Federal Truth in Lending law. When a patient offers to compromise and make installment payments, it is much better to respond with, "We would prefer you pay whatever sum you can each month until the bill is resolved."

There are those patients who never intend to make a payment for services. There are at least two major reasons for their unwillingness. First, the patient may be disgruntled about the services they received or the size of the bill. When this occurs, it is best to get to the heart of the problem and try to resolve it. Determining the patient's problem or unwillingness to pay can greatly increase the speed of collection.

The second major reason for not receiving payment has little to do with the quality of care received or the size of the bill. The patient simply refuses to make payments for any medical services. No matter how much effort is exerted by the practitioner, little if any money will be collected. Individuals such as these should have their over-due accounts turned over to a collection agency. It is doubtful, however, that the collection agency will meet with much better results than the practitioner.

SETTING A COLLECTION TIMETABLE

Each Practitioner will need to develop a collection timetable so as to follow through on all attempts to collect for patient services. In general, collection attempts will include both telephone and mailing efforts. There should be several attempts by both telephone and mail over a hundred and twenty to one hundred and forty day period.

The Collection Timetable

120-140 Day Schedule

1. Send the patient a statement at the end of thirty days after the services have been provided.

2. At the end of sixty days, send the patient a billing statement along with a short letter. (Letter One: "We have yet to receive any response from you concerning our previous billing attempts. Please contact the office as soon as possible.")

3. Seventy-five days. Telephone Call One: Make sure your assistant reaches the patient. Express concern for the lack of payment. Ask how soon the practice can expect payment. Document the response.

4. Ninety days. Send another statement along with another reminder. (Letter Two: "We have yet to hear from you regarding the over-due account. Please contact us as soon as possible. Let us know when we can expect payment.")

5. One hundred and five days. Telephone Call Two: Continue to express concern for the patient. Once again, reassure them you are attempting to be cooperative. Encourage them to promise a date of payment.

6. One hundred and twenty days. Send a third and final letter along with another billing statement. (Letter Three: "We expect full payment for services on the over-due account. If you do not contact the office within ten days and arrange payment, we will be forced to seek another course of action to secure payment.")

7. Give the patient a period of time to respond. If no payment or phone call is received by day one hundred and forty, turn the account over to a collection agency. You have done everything you can.

USING A COLLECTION AGENCY OR FILING SUIT

A physical therapist should not be reluctant to persue an account that becomes over-due. When all attempts to collect for services fail, the question often becomes one of should the practitioner use a collection agency or sue for payment?

Collection agencies are widely used by many medical professionals. A good collection agency can often motivate an individual to make payments on an over-due account that were previously unsuccessful. The average fee for collecting on medical services is 50 percent. Most reputable collection agencies will require one-half of all the money that is collected.

Once you threaten to use a collection agency you must follow through or possibly be in violation of federal collection statutes. The failure to follow through also helps to lower your credibility. Before choosing a collection agency check with members of the local medical community about the agencies they use and their reliability.

Filing a lawsuit to collect for services can create problems. A patient who believes they were treated wrongfully may file a counter-suit alleging there was malpractice. If you are sure the malpractice possibility does not exist, legal action may quickly stimulate payment.

If you choose to use the legal process to secure payment, many states will allow the case to be filed in small claims court. In these proceedings there is rarely the need for an attorney and filing fees are usually small. In most instances the hearings will take only a few moments.

Once the court date is established, one person (not necessarily the practitioner) must go to court. This person should be prepared to present documentation showing the therapist rendered the services at a reasonable fee. The same individual must also be prepared to negotiate payment. In many cases, the patient will not show up and the practitioner will win by default.

When there are several accounts to be pursued, the court may allow the practitioner to group the claims. To speed up the legal process a court may decide to hear several claims within a specific time period. This helps the legal process operate more smoothly and reduces employee or practitioner time away from the office.

TO PREVENT EMBEZZLEMENT: CHECK THE BOOKS

The temptation for an employee to pocket some of the money which belongs to the practice can sometimes be over-whelming. Embezzlement can occur in all professions but is often easy to accomplish in a small private practice. Embezzlement occurs when an employee willfully keeps some of the money which should have been recorded on the practice books.

Embezzlement schemes can go on for many years without detection. In some cases, an employee is so skilled at the process that the practitioner has no way to assess how much money was lost even after the scheme is uncovered. Embezzlement is, however, easily prevented by simply performing a spot check of the financial records of the practice.

THE MOST COMMON WAYS TO EMBEZZLE

There are primarily three ways in which an employee will attempt to embezzle. Each instance can best be examined through a private practice example. The following present the most common forms of employee embezzlement.

1. **The patient makes a cash payment.** A patient was seen by the physical therapist for a one-week period of treatment. During this time, the treatment services amounted to one hundred twenty-five dollars. On the last visit the patient went to the desk to pay the bill. The patient made a partial cash payment of seventy-five dollars and asked to be billed for the remaining amount. The employee kept the seventy-five dollars and recorded the payment on the patient's ledger card but not on the day sheet. The patient has no way of knowing what transpired since he will still only receive a bill for fifty dollars.

2. **Through the mail.** The employee who is responsible for opening the mail also has the opportunity to keep any cash payments. Once again, if partial payment is received it will not be recorded on the day sheet. If the patient makes a full cash payment through the mail the money can be pocketed and the ledger card destroyed. The employee will destroy the ledger card so the patient will no longer receive a bill.

In rare instances, it is also possible for an employee to open an account in another bank using the practitioners name. The employee will then periodically deposit checks into the account after carefully recording the amount on the ledger card but not on the day sheet.

3. **Altering accounts payable.** This method is not very common but may occur. In situations such as these an assistant will make out checks with an erasable ink pen. After the practitioner signs the checks, the assistant alters to whom the check is made payable. The amount paid can also be altered since the assistant has complete access to the financial records, and knows how to balance the payments. The assistant is rarely discovered because the checks and bank statements are returned to the office where they can be destroyed. The only time methods such as these are discovered is when the accountant carefully reviews the books or the practitioner receives threatening letters for nonpayment.

HOW TO DETERMINE THERE IS A PROBLEM

There are many ways for an employee to alter records in order to embezzle money. People who attempt to embezzle operate from the belief that they are smarter than the practitioner and can beat the system. This assumption is false when the practitioner knows some of the most common signs of employee embezzlement.

Things to Look For:

1. Patients complain about errors in their monthly statements.
2. Payments to the practice remain constant rather than showing normal business fluctuations.
3. Drops in practice income, not consistant with patient volume.
4. An employee refuses to take a vacation for fear of having financial record changes discovered.
5. Employee's lifestyle is beyond what the salary should indicate.
6. Records are rewritten so as to look neater.
7. Practice business patterns change when a certain employee is absent.

Prevention Is the Key

The practitioner who maintains tight internal control will stand a better chance is safeguarding against embezzlement. The practitioner should know each employee well enough so as to detect any personality changes or financial difficulties. Make the employees feel as though they can come to you in confidence to discuss any personal problems. In general, the most common methods to prevention include:

1. **Closely follow the bank statements each month.** Practice mail may be addressed to a post office box rather than being sent to the office. The practitioner may wish to go and personally collect the mail rather than delegate this responsibility. A record should be maintained by the person opening the mail of each check and cash payment received. The person opening the mail should not be the same person who does the actual posting on the financial records.

2. **Allow no one else to sign checks.** The signing of checks should not be delegated to an employee unless absolutely necessary. The preparation of the payroll and the actual paying of the employees should be done by two different individuals. Neither the owner nor the person authorized to do so should ever sign a blank check.

3. **Have all checks stamped, "for deposit only."** The practitioner should either personally make the daily bank deposits or compare the bank deposits made against the record of cash and checks received. There should always be a duplicate copy of the bank deposit or other documentation from the bank insuring the money was deposited. If the practitioner delegates these jobs there must be a periodic check of performance.

When using a computer make sure the programming will reveal any unauthorized use or evidence of program alterations or tampering. Entering false data may be one way to attempt computer embezzlement. Many problems with computer embezzlement can be prevented through minimizing the after hours use of the computer and periodically monitoring all inputs and outputs.

CHAPTER TEN

THE ESSENTIAL MANAGERIAL FUNCTIONS
OF PRIVATE PRACTICE

THE OWNER of a private practice has a demanding job. As a practitioner, you are responsible for employee morale, motivation, development, and leadership. In order for the practice to be successful, you must have considerable knowledge about the managerial aspects of supervision and the behavioral factors that help motivate employees. Above everything else, your actions must ultimately reflect the welfare of each and every patient.

As a private practitioner, you soon discover there is a dual role of responsibility. You are not only a medical professional who cares for patients on a daily basis, but also a business professional. It is therefore essential that you conduct your affairs and provide medical care as effectively as any person would in another area of business.

In any practice situation there should be a working atmosphere where employees receive as much satisfaction from their jobs as possible. A properly managed practice will allow employees to satisfy their individual needs for achievement and recognition. The more satisfied employees are with their working environment, the more likely they are to work towards practice goals and assume greater responsibility in patient care.

THE MANAGER AND PRACTITIONER

It is important to understand the two types of work a physical therapist/manager performs. First, there is the physical therapy services you provide as a health care professional. These are primarily concerned with patient treatment. These functions include the treatment methods, techniques, and equipment involved in the rehabilitation of a patient.

The second type of work is practice management. Management in a private practice is the ability to accomplish objectives by directing the practice personnel toward common objectives and goals. Management work involves the five activities of planning, organizing, staffing, controlling, and influencing. Every individual who acts in a managerial capacity must perform, at least to some degree, these processes of management; quite often simultaneously. How effectively a single managerial process is accomplished will ultimately affect how the other processes are performed.

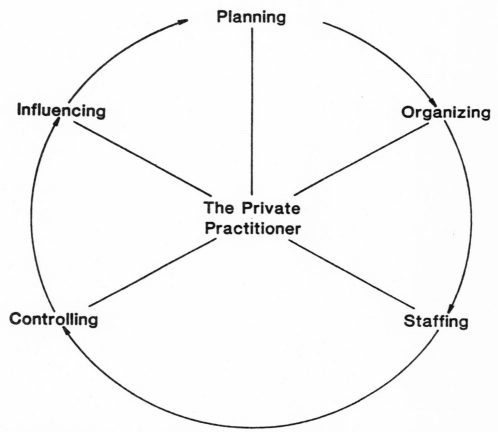

Figure XXXII. The five managerial functions of the private practitioner. Practice success requires some part of each day will be devoted to performing each of these functions.

The Managerial Functions: Planning

Planning is the managerial task that determines in advance, what activities are to be performed by the practice. Planning consists of defining the practice mission and purpose as well as determining the objectives, policies, procedures, and methods of practice organization.

For many, planning is the most difficult of the five managerial functions. Planning is intellectual work involving the determination of what the practice will do in the future. When you plan, you set the practice direction.

Planning must come before any of the other managerial functions. The techniques and methods used to develop plans will directly affect how the other managerial processes are carried out. The decisions made during the intellectual planning process will provide the other functions with objectives and standards of performance.

One of the primary benefits of planning in a private practice is that it clearly defines the purpose and goals of the practice. It provides a basis for unified action by all employees, thereby reducing the risk of practice failure.

Planning also contributes to the development of a more favorable human relations climate. Employees are more likely to be assigned jobs where they can contribute and gain more satisfaction from their work. Many potential personnel problems can be avoided, or at least minimized, by proper planning.

The Planning Process in Private Practice:

1. Develop a practice objective. The first step in planning is to develop a practice objective. The practice objective strategically identifies the direction in which the practice is to proceed. Every employee should be familiar with the practice objective statement. It outlines the end result toward which all practice activities will be directed. For example, the objective of this practice is to provide high quality rehabilitation, at the lowest possible cost to the patient, while ensuring a profitable practice.

2. Secondary objective. Once the primary practice objective has been established, there may also be a need to develop other or secondary objectives. Secondary objectives are much narrower in scope. The purpose of secondary objectives is to allow an even greater focus on the direction, growth, and development in the practice. Examples are: (a) to increase public awareness of physical therapy and the services which are offered by the practice, (b) to provide a practice environment that allows each employee to best utilize their training and experience while achieving personal satisfaction from employment at the facility, (c) provide opportunities for employees to attend continuing education seminars and encourage the application of procedures and methods learned into patient treatment.

After establishing the objectives for the practice, it is essential to develop additional plans to allow for their implementation. These plans include the formulation of policies, procedures, methods, rules, and budgets. All of these work together in a coordinated fashion to allow the practice objectives to be accomplished.

POLICIES

Closely related to the objectives of the practice are the policies. Policies guide actions that are necessary to achieve objectives. Policies are general guides to thinking. They help provide the individual employee who has a decision making responsibility with a direction to assist in the final decision. Objectives determine what is to be done and policies determine how it will be done.

Policies are essential in private practice. Employees are sensitive to any differences in supervisory treatment. Demonstrated favoritism by a practitioner when making decisions can quickly destroy morale in a private practice. A policy should serve to reassure all employees that they will be treated fairly and objectively. Policies should allow the employee to consistantly know what to expect from an employer.

All policies should be communicated to those employees in the practice to whom they apply. They should be in writing and explained to individual employees whenever questions arise. The managerial process of actually writing policies is very time consuming but does provide benefits. Whenever needed, the individual employee has an easy reference point which will guide decision making and action. Policies are also helpful to new employees in explaining how the practice operates.

Policies Should Be Flexible

The primary purpose of a policy is to assist in keeping an employee aimed in the right direction. They should be defined as broad guidelines to thinking. They can, however, be flexible and contain words such as "whenever possible."

Policies should exist to aid in the delegation of responsibility to employees. They approve, in advance, the decisions made by employees as long as they are made within the boundaries of the policy. This should make the role of practice manager much easier. Once you have properly defined the policies for the practice, you can feel reasonably confident that the employees will make decisions within the prescribed limits. In order for this to work, policies must be explicitly stated and communicated to those employees in the practice to whom they are to apply.

RULES

A rule is unlike a policy, procedure, or method. Rules are activities you do not want employees engaged in while at work. They provide guides to inaction rather than action. Some examples include; "no smoking" or "no eating."

There will be instances when the practitioner has to set down specific guidelines for appropriate behavior. Do not establish rules in an arbitrary fashion. Always explain each rule and clarify the various ways the employees could become involved in an offense before it happens.

BUDGETS

Objectives, policies, procedures, and methods can only be meaningful if they are supported financially through a budget. Budgets are plans that express anticipated results in terms of money, employee man hours, equipment needs, and potential practice growth and expansion. Budgeting is vital to private practice survival.

The budget is an example of a plan that is designed to be used only once. It is a guide to be used during the period of time in which it was intended. After that period of time, whether it be one month or a year, it will not be called upon again. A new planning period must be developed and a new budget established.

A budget is a plan that is expressed in numbers. The advantage of budget development is that it will state objectives in specifics rather than generalities. The figures stated in the budget will allow the immediate assessment of whether objectives and goals are being achieved. Budgets are not merely forecasts, but are to be standards by which the daily operation of the practice functions. It is essential that the private practitioner stay within the guidelines of the budget to ensure the economic success of the practice.

PRIVATE PRACTICE BUDGETING

Budget development need not be difficult. The primary purpose is to allow the immediate assessment of the financial health of the practice. Budgets can be developed for a single month or for an entire year. Practice objectives and goals determine the length of time chosen.

The following is an example of one of the simplest forms of practice budgets. It can be used to assess the practice on a month to month basis and also review at year's end.

PRIVATE PRACTICE BUDGET

	JAN	FEB	MAR	APR	MAY	JUNE	TOTALS	JULY	AUG	SEPT	OCT	NOV	DEC	TOTALS	YEAR TO DATE
TREATMENTS	125	135	175	165	185	191	976	325	300	325	400	400	400	2150	3126
AVERAGE FEE - $25.00															
COLLECTED FEES	3125	3375	4375	4125	4625	4775	24,400	8125	7500	8125	10,000	10,000	10,000	53,750	78,150
	2500	2700	3500	3300	3700	3820	19,520	6500	6000	6500	8000	8000	8000	43,000	62,520
EXPENSES															
1. Advertising & Promotion	200	100	100	75	50	50	575	-0-	-0-	25	50	75	-0-	150	725
2. Dues & Subscriptions	20	20	20	20	20	20	120	20	20	20	20	20	20	120	240
3. Educational Expenses	60	60	60	60	60	60	360	60	60	60	60	60	60	360	720
4. Insurance	800	800	800	800	800	800	4800	800	800	800	800	800	800	4800	9,600
5. Laundry	75	75	75	75	75	75	450	75	75	75	75	75	75	450	900
6. Legal & Audit	100	100	100	100	100	100	600	100	100	100	100	100	100	600	1,200
7. Salaries															
a) Physical Therapists	2000	2000	2000	2000	2000	2000	12,000	2000	2000	2000	2000	2000	2000	12,000	24,000
b) Aide	-0-	-0-	-0-	-0-	-0-	-0-	-0-	-0-	-0-	-0-	1800	1800	1800	5,400	5,400
c) Sec/Rec	1000	1000	1000	1000	1000	1000	6,000	1000	1000	1000	1000	1000	1000	6,000	12,000
8. Office Expenses	100	100	100	100	150	150	700	150	150	150	200	200	200	1,050	1,750
9. Equipment Lease	150	150	150	150	150	150	900	150	150	150	150	150	150	900	1,800
10. Professional Supplies	25	25	25	25	25	25	150	25	25	25	25	25	25	150	300
11. Payroll Taxes	300	300	300	300	300	300	1,800	300	300	300	400	400	400	2,100	3,900
12. Rent & Parking	1000	1000	1000	1000	1000	1000	6,000	1000	1000	1000	1000	1000	1000	6,000	12,000
13. Repair & Maintenance	-0-	-0-	50	50	-0-	50	100	-0-	-0-	100	-0-	-0-	50	150	250
14. Taxes & License	75	75	75	75	75	75	450	75	75	75	75	75	75	450	900
15. Telephone	100	100	100	100	100	100	600	100	100	100	100	100	100	600	1,200
16. Utilities	200	200	200	200	200	200	1,200	200	200	200	200	200	200	1,200	2,400
TOTAL EXPENSES	6205	6105	6105	6130	6105	6155	36,805	6055	6055	6180	8055	8080	8055	42,480	79,285
PROFIT (LOSS) (1)	3080	(2730)	(1730)	2005	(1480)	(1380)	(2,405)	2070	1445	1945	1945	1920	1945	11,270	(1,135)
PROFIT (LOSS) (2)	(3705)	(3405)	(2605)	(2830)	(2405)	(2335)	(17,285)	445	(55)	320	(55)	(80)	(55)	520	(16,765)

The importance of cash collections cannot be overemphasized.
This budget projects only an 80% collection rate during the
first year of operation. From this projection it is estimated that
the practice will sustain a $16,765 loss.

	1st 6 MONTHS	2nd 6 MONTHS	YEAR TO DATE
PROFIT (LOSS) ACCRUAL BASIS	(2,405)	11,270	(1,135)
PROFIT (LOSS) CASH BASIS	(17,285)	520	(16,765)

Figure XXXIII.

HOW THE BUDGET WORKS

First: Determine the Income

1. Estimate the approximate number of patients the practice will treat each month.

2. Determine the average fee to be charged to each patient.

3. Multiply the average fee times the estimated number of monthly treatments. This figure represents the projected monthly income. The projected monthly income figure will be on the accrual basis, not on the collected basis. This figure represents what the practice could make if every patient paid their entire bill. This is seldom the case. A good collection rate for most practices is ninety percent.

4. By multiplying the projected monthly income times the anticipated collection rate, you can determine what the estimated income will be.

Second: Determine Expenses

The Fifteen Major Areas

1. **Advertising.** Announcements to the local practitioners and the printing of business cards.

2. **Dues and Subscriptions.** Includes professional dues as well as magazines for the waiting room.

3. **Travel.** Money alloted for travel to state and national conventions.

4. **Insurance.** Malpractice, liability, life, health, accident, disability, and workers' compensation.

5. **Laundry.** Towels, pillowcases, sheets, etc.

6. **Legal.** Attorney and accounting services.

7. **Salaries.** Both professional and nonprofessional.

8. **Payroll Expenses.** These are generally paid on a quarterly basis. They are determined as a percentage of the total wages paid. The Internal Revenue Service or a local accountant can provide the necessary forms.

9. **Rent or Lease Property.**

10. **Repair and Maintenance of Equipment.**

11. **Office Supplies and Furniture.** Leased or purchased.

12. **Professional Supplies.** Creams, jells, alcohol, etc.

13. **Taxes and Licenses.** Occupational and business licenses as well as state and local taxes.

14. **Telephone.**

15. **Utilities.**

PROJECTING PRACTICE PROFIT OR LOSS

There are two items to look at to determine whether the practice is making a profit or incurring a loss. Examine both the accrual basis and the cash basis.

Accrual Basis

Subtract the total projected expenses from the total projected earned fees. This figure (1) represents how much the practice has "accrued." The accrual figure may not be considered realistic. It assumes a 100 percent collection rate. It does, however, allow you to determine whether the practice is seeing enough patients to afford continued operation under present conditions.

Cash Basis

Subtract the total projected expenses from the total fees collected. This is a more realistic figure (2) since it indicates whether the practice is acquiring enough revenue to cover expenses.

ORGANIZING

The managerial process of organizing defines the organizational structure of the practice. To organize is to design a structural framework which defines all the employee relationships that are needed to provide medical care.

Organizing automatically follows planning since it determines what practice members are going to do to accomplish objectives. Organizing involves defining the duties, authority, responsibilities, and relationships of each employee in the practice.

There are many types of organizational structure. In the hospital setting, the functional type of structure is most common. Here, the practice is to group those who perform the same function in one area. Examples of these are the dietary department, the department of human resources, and the department of radiology.

In private practice, the most prevalent type of organization is the line structure. The line structure, sometimes called the scalar structure, is the oldest and simplest type of structure. It demonstrates a clear line of authority is to be maintained from the highest to the lowest level within the practice. Each employee in the practice is held directly responsible to only one superior. Being responsible to only one superior is known as the unity of command principle.

Unity of command means that there is only one person at each level in the practice who has the authority to make a decision appropriate to that position. Each employee has a single immediate supervisor up and down the chain of command. Under this form of organization, each employee knows who their immediate supervisor is and who can give them instructions.

ESTABLISHING A FORMAL ORGANIZATIONAL CHART

An organizational chart is a graphical means of portraying the practice structure. The chart shows the relationships and groupings of employee functions.

ORGANIZATIONAL STRUCTURE

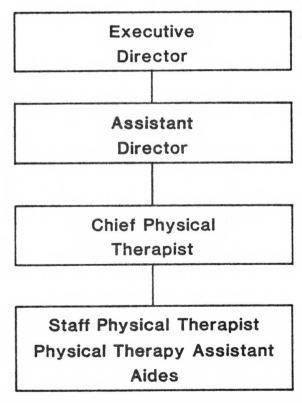

Figure XXXIV. One of the primary advantages of this type of practice structure is that it can easily be read and understood. The organizational chart is designed for unity of command.

Organizational charts begin with the representation of a number of boxes that are interconnected. The boxes are interconnected to demonstrate the grouping of activities which make up a practice. The ability to determine who reports to whom is by noting how the boxes are related to one another in a scalar relationship.

JOB DESCRIPTIONS/JOB SPECIFICATIONS

Job descriptions objectively describe the elements of a position. They indicate the duties and functions required by an employee. Job specifications indicate the human qualities necessary to perform the job safely and adequately. Job specifications include the education, training, and experience required to hold the position.

Job descriptions can prove invaluable to the practitioner. They can be used to help the practitioner in the interview and selection of potential employees. For new employees, they can be a guide in determining what activities should be performed on the job. The job description can also be used to evaluate and appraise individual employee performance.

STAFFING

Staffing a practice involves the process of analyzing present and future employee needs and obtaining qualified individuals to meet those needs. The staffing function involves the recruitment, selection, placement, development, training, and compensation of the employees of a practice. It is the practitioners responsibility to evaluate and appraise the performance of employees, to promote them according to demonstrated competence, to reward them and when necessary, to discipline and possibly discharge them. To properly perform the staffing function, the practitioner must fulfill all of these duties.

The importance of the staffing function cannot be overemphasized. The employees of the practice serve a vital public relations role. They are the first to greet patients, and convey the philosophy of the practice. How well they do this can either win or lose patients.

Many practitioners see only the professional competence of the staff person as it relates to the delivery of physical therapy. When patients stop coming to the office, the practitioner usually blames the practice decline on an increasing number of facilities offering out-patient physical therapy. In many cases, the reality is more likely to be an abrupt handling of patients by practice employees.

In private practice, the staffing function is a continuous activity. It is not something that is only to be performed when first opening an office. Sound managerial principles indicate the importance to the practitioner's involvement in the interview and selection of employees. This process should not be delegated to someone else. Only by participating in the actual interview and selection process can the practitioner be assured that the best employees are chosen to provide health care.

INFLUENCING

The influencing function is the managerial process whereby the practitioner evokes action from employees in order to accomplish practice objectives. Influencing in health care can also be known as motivating, directing, or actuating. Regardless of the terminology, it is the managerial function which attempts to gain maximum employee performance while providing a working environment which allows the employee to find personal satisfaction. This function includes problems with employee motivation, the issuance of directives, and overseeing employee guidance.

There are many variables which may potentially influence the motivational level of the staff. Some variables can be controlled by the practitioner while others cannot. In a private practice there are a minimum of five variables you should closely examine to enhance the atmosphere of the practice.

Be a Manager

Employees of the practice look to the owner for guidance and decision making ability. Management leadership is responsible for establishing the practice climate which enhances motivation. The manager must be comfortable with the idea that his or her role is to influence outcomes, communicate changes to employees, and set an example of how to get things done. The more aware the practitioner is of the ability to influence outcomes, the greater the potential to achieve practice objectives.

Communication

The practice manager must exhibit an ability to clearly define what is expected of employees. Staff members should know what constitutes acceptable and unacceptable levels of patient care. Demonstrate how patient care can be improved, and follow up to see if results are being obtained. Encourage employees to "live up to the quality of care" as outlined in practice objectives.

Do not overlook the area of job descriptions. Never assume that a job description discussed in the selection interview will provide enough guidance to a new employee. In many instances, job descriptions are not specific enough or the employee was too nervous to recall everything that was discussed. Once hired, review again what is expected.

Managerial Feedback

It is the practitioner's responsibility to inform employees whether or not their assigned tasks are being performed correctly. Feedback concerning job performance should be provided for both positive and negative forms of employee behavior. Employees cannot offer the quality of health care desired unless expectations are communicated to them.

In many practice situations, feedback is only provided on an annual or semiannual basis. Feedback is usually incorporated into the performance evaluation prior to awarding or denying a merit raise. Provide employees with feedback as frequently as possible. Take a few moments to recognize individual or group performance by thanking the staff for a job well done during a particularly busy week. Inform individual staff members about positive comments which patients communicated regarding their performance.

Provide negative feedback in a manner which avoids embarrassing the employee. Do not criticize performance in front of other employees. Instead, do so in the privacy of an office. Do not continually stress the problem, but rather indicate to the employee that you recognize there is a problem and offer to assist in taking action to correct the unwanted behavior.

Employee Goal Setting

The private practitioner's primary goal is to always offer the highest quality medical care to the patient. This goal sets the general direction for the practice. It can, however, be further enhanced by allowing employees to also participate in practice goal development.

Employees can be asked to develop individual goals they would like to see accomplished by the practice. Goals can be developed which will make the operations and functions of the practice more profitable but do not detract from providing high quality patient care.

Goals, such as reducing waiting room time for patients through more efficient scheduling, encourage employee committment and provides for a more satisfied group of patients. Assist the employee in goal development, check the level of performance, and allow flexibility in establishing a time frame for assessing goal attainment.

Be Accessible: Meet Regularly with the Staff

In any private medical practice, regular monthly staff meetings are a must. Meetings can be on a one-to-one basis or they can involve the entire staff. Regardless of the design, the primary goal of staff meetings is to increase communication among the members of the practice. Communication is vital not only for the purpose of social satisfaction but also to attain effective job performance.

In an established practice, there should be at least one monthly staff meeting with required attendance by all employees. In a new or rapidly growing practice, it may be necessary to conduct one or more weekly staff meetings to keep employees fully informed of changing conditions.

Every effort should be made to make all meetings informal and relaxed. Try to provide a relaxed atmosphere for questions to be asked and answered. Meetings should not be abandoned once the practice becomes successful. Too often, meetings go by the wayside once the patient volume increases. Many problems with motivation can be avoided if the practitioner demonstrates an eagerness to meet with and listen to employee suggestions and comments.

When not conducting meetings, try to maintain an open door policy. This is a less formal approach of encouraging individual employees to come talk with you in the privacy of your office. The open door policy is an effort to further maintain open lines of communication between the practitioner and employees.

It is not a requirement that you become extremely friendly with employees in order to have a successful medical office. It is more important, however, that you listen to their problems, periodically express warmth and appreciation for their efforts, and sincerely attempt to provide a good working atmosphere.

CONTROLLING

Controlling is the managerial function of reviewing and measuring performance in order to determine the extent to which practice plans and objectives are being achieved. Controlling provides the practitioner with a basis for detecting and correcting deviations from plans and objectives.

The controlling process is very closely related to the other managerial functions of planning. When the manager of a practice sets goals, objectives, and policies they become standards against which performance is appraised. If performance does not meet with standards, then corrective action must be taken.

To perform the controlling function in private practice, there are three steps which should be followed.

1. The practitioner sets practice standards.
2. There is a check of performance.
3. Take corrective action.

Practice Standards

Controlling assumes the existence of established objectives and goals. The objectives or goals developed in the planning process constitute the standards to be employed in the controlling process.

Check of Performance

Once standards have been developed, there must be a check to see if actual performance meets with the standards. Reviewing performance is usually done after the actual activity has been performed.

There are two ways the practitioner can check to determine performance compliance. Performance can be ascertained by either checking the actual work or by studying prepared reports. Information contained in the reports is then compared with preset standards of performance.

Corrective Action

Control is not limited to only the measurement of performance and the analysis of reports. Action is required when it is determined that there are weaknesses or mistakes. The urgency of action required depends upon the nature of the situation.

In some instances, it may be determined that the deviation from the performance standard is related to an employee who was not given proper directions. Situations such as these are simple to correct. The practitioner once again explains the standards which are to be followed.

BUDGETING AS A CONTROLLING DEVICE

The budget may be one of the most important controlling devices to the practitioner. It is essential that every private practitioner learn how to project budgets, live within their boundries, and use them properly for controlling purposes.

Developing the budget is part of the planning function but its actual administration is part of the controlling function. Budgets are standards by which the actual operations of the practice are to be compared. The budget reflects actual performance against the plan. This enables the practitioner to take corrective action.

In most instances, budgets state anticipated results in numerical terms. There are, however, budgets which can indicate the number of staff members needed and the number of man-hours required. However used, the planning of a budget sets the standards of achievement. The control function allows the practitioner to determine the level of compliance and the corrective action, if any, that is needed.

THE MANAGERIAL FUNCTIONS ARE INSEPARABLE

The five managerial functions of the private practitioner are inseparable. Each function interrelates and influences the other functions. If the practitioner does not perform all of the managerial functions to a certain extent, the practice can never reach its maximum potential.

It is not feasible for any practitioner to set aside a specific amount of time each day to perform a given function. The time spent on each function will vary as practice conditions and circumstances change. There is little doubt that the planning function must come first in any private practice. Without well developed plans, the practitioner cannot organize, staff, influence, or control.

SAMPLE POLICIES
AND PROCEDURES MANUAL

The following is to be used only as a **guide** to actual manual preparation. The policies and procedures provided are **not inclusive** nor are they recommended for all practice settings.

INTRODUCTION

The information contained in this organizational manual is to be used as a guide by practice members. The objectives and goals as outlined represent what is believed to be the highest performance and the maximum in physical therapy relating to any set of circumstances.

It is the intention of the management of this practice that the material contained within this manual is to be used in a consultative manner. It is understood that individual circumstances may arise which require modification of the policies and procedures as presented.

SUBJECT

Purpose of Anytown Physical Therapy Clinic

Effective Date: 1/1/XX

POLICY

The purpose of the Anytown Physical Therapy Clinic is to provide rehabilitative services to those individuals who have chronic and acute disabilities and/or injuries. Physical therapists will provide their services to patients on the referral and/or prescription of a physician as outlined by the laws of this state.

The practice of physical therapy is directed towards assisting individuals who present disability, pain, and/or decreased motor skills. Attempts will be made to reduce further disability, relieve pain, and restore function within individual patient capabilities.

The management of Anytown Physical Therapy Clinic will revise the statement of purpose and the organizational plan as needed. A complete review of this manual will be conducted annually and a report made to all employees.

SUBJECT

Personnel Qualifications and Practice Hours of Operations

Effective Date: 1/1/XX

The Anytown Physical Therapy Clinic is under the direction of a licensed/ registered physical therapist. Additional professional and supportive personnel will also be present to assist in patient care.

HOURS OF OPERATION

1. The practice will be open Monday thru Friday; 8:00 A.M. to 5:00 P.M.
2. Weekend hours provided upon individual request.

STAFFING

1. Title of practice manager is Director of Physical Therapy.
2. Nonadministrative personnel include: two physical therapists, one physical therapy assistant, three physical therapy aides, and one receptionist.
3. Staffing plans provide for one physical therapist to be assisted by a one or two assistant/aide team. Patient volume will maintain a maximum of eighteen to twenty-two patient visits per day per physical therapist.

QUALIFICATIONS

Physical therapists and physical therapy assistants are to be graduates of a physical therapy program recognized by the American Physical Therapy Association. Physical therapists and physical therapy assistants must possess and maintain licensure according to the laws of the state. Both professionals must maintain adequate medical malpractice insurance.

The owner/manager of Anytown Physical Therapy Clinic is to act in a supervisory capacity. It is the owner/manager's responsibility to participate in programs of employee education and administration.

Physical therapy aides are to receive on-the-job training following all guidelines and recommendations provided by the American Physical Therapy Association. They are to provide patient care only under the direct supervision of a physical therapist or physical therapy assistant.

SUBJECT

Organizational Plan

Effective Date: 1/1/XX

POLICY

The owner/manager of Anytown Physical Therapy Clinic is responsible for the organization, administration, and supervision of physical therapy services. The manager will act in a manner that facilitates maximum ethical and professional standards in health care.

The owner/manager is responsible for the direction and supervision of personnel in accordance with the policies established within this manual. The supervisor is to maintain coordination and cooperation with other providers of health care in the community.

Positions and job responsibilities described in this manual are established for physical therapists, physical therapy assistants, and physical therapy aides. Organizational plans and developments will be discussed at monthly staff meetings. Organization charts are available to all employees of the practice.

The organizational chart is provided to assist employees in the delivery of health care. The primary purpose of the chart is to provide effective communication and delegation of all job responsibilities. It is understood that situations or circumstances may arise which would require modification of the organizational chart. The owner/manager will retain responsibility for the performance evaluation of all employees.

Anytown Physical Therapy Clinic
Organizational Chart

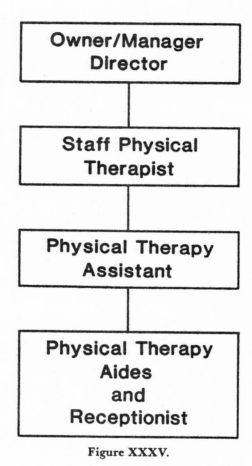

Figure XXXV.

SUBJECT

Equipment

Effective Date: 1/1/XX

POLICY

Equipment is to be provided which will allow employees to offer high quality patient care in a safe and effective manner.

1. Equipment available includes:
   (a) Deepheat
       Ultrasound, two units.
       Diathermy, one unit.
   (b) Superficial heat
       Paraffin bath, one unit.
       Hydrocollators (hotpacks), two units.
   (c) Hydrotherapy
       Low boy whirlpool, one unit.
       Combination leg and arm whirlpool, two units.
   (d) Electrical Stimulation
       Electrogalvanic stimulator, three units.
       Transcutaneous electrical nerve stimulators, four units.
   (e) Traction
       Motorized traction units, two units.
   (f) Gymnasium
       Isokinetic equipment, one unit.
       Continuous passive motion, one unit.
       Wall pulley set, one unit.
       Parallel bar, one unit.
       Set metal weights, one unit.
       Set sand bags, one unit.
       Wheelchair, one unit.
2. Replacement and purchase of new equipment will be assessed and budgeted on an annual basis.
3. All physical therapy equipment is under a program of preventive maintenance. Calibration and safety inspections are to be performed on an annual basis.
4. New equipment is to be inspected and tested prior to patient use.

SUBJECT

Care of Physical Therapy Equipment

Effective Date: 1/1/XX

POLICY

1. Shortwave Diathermy
   (a) Inspect unit before each patient treatment.
   (b) Report any defective equipment to the director immediately. Do not use defective equipment.
   (c) Check all connections.
   (d) All manual adjustments should be in working order and secure.
   (e) Inspect unit for frayed cords, cables, and defective electrodes.
   (f) Check for proper grounding.
   (g) Clean all dials and the surface of the machine weekly.
   (h) All protective coverings should be washed weekly with mild soap and tepid water.
2. Ultrasound
   (a) Follow steps A-H as indicated on shortwave diathermy.
   (b) Clean transducer face following each patient treatment. Alcohol should be applied to the transducer to insure cleanliness and sterility.
3. Traction Units
   (a) Follow steps A-G as indicated on shortwave diathermy.
   (b) Do not use frayed rope or cable.
   (c) Inspect head-halter and straps before each treatment.
4. Electrical Stimulator
   (a) Follow steps A-H as indicated on shortwave diathermy.
   (b) Allow electrode sponges to dry after each treatment.
   (c) Electrodes should be washed monthly.
   (d) Inspect electrodes for corrosion.
5. Paraffin Unit
   (a) Paraffin bath should be sterilized once a month and cleaned regularly to remove any collected sediment.
   (b) Unplug the unit when preparing for patient treatment.
   (c) Unplug the unit when preparing to clean.
   (d) Do not attempt to pour out paraffin.
      1. Dip out paraffin into another large container.
      2. Allow remaining paraffin to solidify.
      3. Gently scrape and remove remaining paraffin.
      4. Wipe out inside of unit with warm water and mild soap.
      5. Refill unit with new paraffin mixture.

6. Hydrocollater
   (a) Clean unit once a month.
   (b) Unplug unit prior to cleaning.
   (c) Drain unit and remove hot packs.
   (d) Clean tank with mild disinfectant or soap. Refill with distilled water.
   (e) Plug in unit after cleaning.
7. Transcutaneous Nerve Stimulator
   (a) Alcohol may be used to remove stains or adhesives from surface of unit.
   (b) Do not immerse unit in water, or use strong solvents to clean unit.
   (c) Wash electrodes with warm water and mild soap after each usage.
   (d) Inspect lead wires for damage to the internal conductor.
8. Emergency Medical Situation
   An emergency medical kit is maintained in the clinic. All employees are to be trained in basic emergency procedures and be cardiopulmonary resuscitation (CPR) certified.
9. Educational Equipment
   To be obtained as needed for in-service presentations.
10. Whirlpool
    (a) After each patient treatment:
        1. All water is to be drained or pumped from the whirlpool.
        2. Rinse tub.
        3. Close drain and refill whirlpool to a level which will permit agitator to operate. Use two ounces of disinfectant and pump this mixture through agitator for three minutes. Drain whirlpool and scrub tank with disinfectant. When finished, thoroughly rinse.
    (b) Sterilizing
        1. To be performed weekly as needed or when presented with a patient who has staph, pseudomonas, or any known bacterial infection.
        2. Complete general procedure for whirlpool care (see above).
        3. Refill tank and add two cups of bleach. Allow agitator to operate ten minutes. When possible, allow water to stand overnight.
        4. At least quarterly, dismantle agitator unit and clean with disinfectant.
11. Procedure for Infection Control
    Each month, the drains and rims of the whirlpools are to be swabbed with a culturette. The culture is to be analyzed by a local lab. Results will be recorded in the infection control log.

SUBJECT

Practice Operating Procedures

Effective Date: 1/1/XX

POLICY

Procedures for management of Anytown Physical Therapy Clinic are developed to help obtain goals as established in the statement of purpose.

Procedures

1. Job descriptions are provided in this section of the policy and procedures manual.
2. Patient scheduling procedures:
    (a) Appointments are to be made directly with the practice via telephone and/or referral. Appointments should be made via telephone prior to the patient's first visit to ensure patients arrive on a scheduled basis.
    (b) Patient treatment orders may be written or obtained by a physician's verbal order. Verbal orders must be followed by written confirmation. Upon receipt of the referral the patient's name, diagnosis, type of treatment, and physician's name are entered into a permanent record book kept by the receptionist. The therapist to whom the patient has been assigned for treatment takes the order and evaluates the recommended treatment. The receptionist then prepares a patient folder entering the patient's name, diagnosis, chart number, treatment, and referring physician. The patient will be asked to fill out a patient information sheet and the method of payment will be established.
    (c) Scheduling is the responsibility of the physical therapy director and the receptionist.
    (d) The patient is interviewed by the therapist. The interview should include the following:
    1. Subjective information regarding the disease or injury.
    2. Objective information provided by records, test information, or evaluation by the physical therapist.
    3. Assess the patient status and select a plan of care within the parameters of the referral and as defined by the state physical therapy practice act.
    (e) When objective findings are not consistant with recommended treatment, it is the physical therapist's responsibility to contact the referring physician to discuss findings and offer recommendations.
    (f) Procedure for preparing the patient schedule. Using the previous day's schedule and preceding week's schedule, a daily schedule will be developed for patient treatment. A schedule will also be developed for the following day and subsequent week. All employees will be advised of the daily schedule and any changes.

(g) Patients for consult are to have a plan of care developed by the physical therapist as indicated by the problem-oriented record system. The plan of care is to be approved by the physician. The plan of care may be mailed to the physician for signature along with a self-addressed stamped envelope.

3. Safety Precautions:
   (a) All electrical equipment is to be grounded.
   (b) Lock brakes on wheelchairs before transferring a patient.
   (c) Footstools, belts, and safety supports are to be used to safely transfer all patients.
   (d) Two persons are to assist in transfers when evaluation of functional status indicates possible difficulty with single transfers.

4. Fire Safety and Evacuation Plans:
   (a) Person(s) discovering the fire is to notify the fire department.
   (b) Safely remove all patients from the practice.
   (c) Unplug equipment, turn off lights, and close doors.
   (d) Perform head count outside of the building to confirm that everyone has been evacuated.

5. Supplies and Equipment:
   (a) All supplies and equipment are to be ordered by the director of physical therapy.
   (b) The director is to be responsible for all equipment. The checking and cleaning of equipment is by established procedure. Calabration of electrical equipment, unless otherwise indicated, will be on an annual basis.
   (c) Laundry service will be provided on a twice weekly basis. Under an established contract, the laundry will be delivered to the clinic on Tuesday and Thursday mornings.

Operational Plans

1. Supervision:
   (a) Title of practice owner: Director of Physical Therapy.
   (b) Other personnel: two physical therapists, one physical therapy assistant, three physical therapy aides and one receptionist.
   (c) Supervisory responsibility according to job title:
   Director of Physical Therapy: Organizing and directing department operation.
   Director of Physical Therapy and Staff Physical Therapist: orientating, instructing, and supervising practice personnel.
   Director of Physical Therapy: scheduling employee working hours and assigning duties.
   Director of Physical Therapy: maintaining and ordering equipment and supplies.
   Director of Physical Therapy, Physical Therapist, Physical Therapy Assistant and Receptionist: maintaining practice records.

2. Personnel Requirements:
   (a) See job descriptions.
   (b) Demonstrate professional attitudes through appearance and performance.
3. Transferring patients. Physical therapy aides are to be trained in the proper technique to use in transferring patients. Each aide will be instructed on the use of safety belts and supports to safely transfer a patient with a disability or injury. Proper bodily mechanics are to be stressed in each transfer.
4. Preparation of equipment:
   (a) Inspection, set-up and preparation of equipment is the responsibility of the therapist or the therapy assistant with the assistance of the physical therapy aide.
   (b) Equipment is to be assembled by the physical therapy aide as indicated by the therapist (See job description of the physical therapy aide).
5. Preparation of Patient for Treatment:
   (a) The physical therapist is to select an appropriate therapy for patient treatment. When the prescription is for specific modalities, the therapist is to use individual knowledge, training, and experience to direct patient treatment. Objective findings not consistant with the diagnosis are to be relayed to the physician. When the referral is a consult, the physical therapist is to evaluate and recommend a plan of care. The plan of care is to be signed by the referring physician.
   (b) Patients may be left momentarily unattended when receiving a physical therapy treatment which does not require constant monitoring. No treatment is to be provided unless a physical therapist or physical therapy assistant is on the premises.
6. Maintaining Patient Records. The writing and charting of patient progress is to be the responsibility of the physical therapist and the physical therapy assistant. Initial evaluation and notation is the responsibility of the physical therapist.

Upon subsequent visits, the physical therapist or the physical therapy assistant is responsible for recording patient treatment and response to treatment. The physical therapist will periodically check the record, make notes, and monitor the response to treatment.

Physical therapy aides are responsible for pulling the daily patient charts. These are to be placed in the order the patients are scheduled to arrive for treatment. All records are to be placed in the individual therapist's file at the charting desk.
7. Patient Charges:
   (a) The physical therapist or physical therapy assistant is responsible for indicating the services rendered on the charge slip. Each charge slip is to be signed.
   (b) Charges are written by the receptionist in accordance with policies and procedures established for billing.
   (c) Charges are based on a unit fee per modality or combination of modalities.
   (d) The receptionist is to record all charges on the patient's ledger card and on the day sheets as indicated by established policies and procedures (see bookkeeping policies and procedures).

(e) The receptionist is responsible for collecting fees from patients as outlined by the established policies and procedures (see bookkeeping policies and procedures).

8. Discharge of Patients:
   (a) At the end of the specified number of treatments, the physical therapist will notify the receptionist that the patient is discharged from physical therapy.
   (b) The physical therapist is responsible for writing a discharge summary. This summary will be typed by the receptionist and mailed to the referring physician.

9. Required Administrative Procedures:
   (a) Annual reports to be completed by the Director of Physical Therapy include:
      1. Development of clinic objectives and goals.
      2. Development of budget.
      3. Job performance evaluation of each employee.
   (b) Monthly meetings to be conducted by Director of Physical Therapy include:
      1. Staff meetings.
      2. Inservices.

POSITION DESCRIPTION – DIRECTOR OF ANYTOWN PHYSICAL THERAPY CLINIC

The director of Anytown Physical Therapy Clinic manages the operation of the facility. Job responsibilities include: supervision of staff, preparation of employee work schedules, participation in conferences, maintenance of equipment, answering correspondance, public education and public relations, communicating with personnel, patients, and patient's family members, assisting in patient treatment, and promoting professional growth.

Major Tasks Include

1. Preparation of schedules related to patient treatment, staffing, statistical records, and preparation of the budget.
2. Guidance of personnel in attitudes and goals.
3. Supervision of treatment procedures.
4. Inspection and repair of equipment.
5. Maintaining correspondance with medical doctors.
6. Providing information to the public regarding the profession of physical therapy.
7. Preparation of training programs for new personnel.
8. Recruitment of professional and nonprofessional personnel.
9. Supervision of housekeeping and clerical staff.
10. Assist in administering patient care.
11. Consulting with a patient or family concerning patient treatment.
12. Attendance at professional association meetings and conferences.

Education, Training, and Experience

Graduation from an accredited school of physical therapy with a master's degree is desirable. Current licensure by State Board of Physical Therapy. Five to ten years of physical therapy experience.

Managerial Traits

1. Aptitude. Verbal ability is required to express ideas, opinions, and views when speaking to groups. Ability to analyze data and prepare reports.
2. Numerical ability. Ability to evaluate statistical data and develop practice budgets.
3. Interests. A preference for contacts with employees and patients. The contacts include organizing and planning, developing staff, and assigning personnel.
4. Temperament. Ability to encourage people and establish support for programs and evaluate job performance through established criteria.
5. Physical demands. Work is sedentary except for limited patient treatment.
6. Job relationships. Workers supervised: All practice staff.

POSITION DESCRIPTION
PHYSICAL THERAPIST

Education

Must be a graduate of a physical therapy program approved by the American Physical Therapy Association. Must be eligible for or possess a license from the state to practice physical therapy.

Major Tasks Include

1. Evaluates and treats disabilities, injuries, and diseases through the use of physical therapy procedures as indicated by physician referral.
2. Responsible for patient care and treatment.
3. Instructs and demonstrates physical therapy procedures to patients and family members.
4. Provides care and proper use of equipment.

Professional Requirements

1. Alterness to detect symptoms of unfavorable responses to treatment.
2. Ability to adjust sensitive equipment and time patient treatments.
3. Maintain an efficient work schedule.
4. Preparation of reports and results concerning patient treatment.

Work to be Performed

The physical therapist treats disorders by one or more of the following methods as prescribed by the physician and approved by the state practice act.
1. Massage.
2. Therapeutic exercise.
3. Hydro therapy.
4. Electro therapy.
5. Related duties which include:
    (a) Maintains patient record of treatment including history, diagnosis by physician, description of treatment, progress notes, discharging summary.
    (b) Instructs personnel and students on methods and objectives of physical therapy.
    (c) Assists in inservice development and presentation.
    (d) Willingness to participate in public relations and activity programs.

Workers Supervised

1. Physical therapy assistants.
2. Physical therapy aides.
3. Clerical personnel.

Physical Therapist Traits

1. Aptitude. Verbal ability needed to supervise supportive personnel.
2. Interests. A preference for working with people and maintaining harmony among workers.
3. Temperaments. Ability to direct and control patient treatment.
4. Physical demands. Extensive walking and standing.

POSITION DESCRIPTION
PHYSICAL THERAPY AIDE

The physical therapy aide is an employee who works under the direct supervision of a physical therapist. The physical therapist is to provide the physical therapy aide with training and guidance for the safe and effective execution of job responsibilities.

Department Operation Duties

1. Follow practice procedures concerning the care and cleaning of equipment and treatment areas.
2. Perform clerical activities which include typing, telephone, reception, and appointments.
3. Maintain inventory of supplies and linen.

Patient Treatment Activities

1. Assists in patient preparation, positioning, and draping.
2. Prepares equipment for patient treatment.
3. Assists patients in functional activities including ambulation and transfers.
4. Provides assistance in the application of selected modalities.
5. Reports any adverse reactions concerning treatment to the physical therapist.

Major Tasks Include

1. Assist patients with dressing.
2. Prepare patient for treatment by assisting patient on and off treatment table.
3. Assist patient in practice of activities as directed by physical therapist. Cautions patients as to proper performance.
4. Maintains cleanliness of treatment areas, (a) sorts and stores linen, (b) makes beds, (c) cleans whirlpools, and (d) maintains adequate supply of materials.
5. Performs routine clerical tasks.
6. Responsibilities include the safety of the patients while providing assistance and maintaining cleanliness of the working area.
7. Knowledge. Must have a working knowledge of physical therapy equipment and its general use in patient care.
8. Skills. Initiative and judgement in providing physical and emotional support for the patient.
9. Mental ability. Must work with the understanding of the legal implications involving errors.
10. Dexterity. Must be gentle and confident in dealing with painful injuries.
11. Experience. Previous experience is helpful but on the job training will be provided.
12. Education. Minimum educational level is high school graduate. Must be cardiopulmonary resuscitation (CPR) certified.

13. Physical demands. Must assist in moving both patients and equipment. Works inside with adequate working conditions. Should encounter no abnormal hazards or risks. Extensive standing and walking required.

14. Characteristics. Energetic, flexible, reliable, willing to accept responsibilities, respects patient's right to privacy, and cheerful.

SUBJECT

Continuing Education

Effective Date: 1/1/XX

POLICY

Provisions will be made to permit physical therapists and physical therapy assistants to attend seminars and to participate in activities of state and local chapters of the American Physical Therapy Association.

1. Professional staff will be paid to attend four days per year of continuing education and/or American Physical Therapy Association activities.
2. Compensation will be provided for enrollment and lodging.

SUBJECT

Orientation to Physical Therapy

Effective Date: 1/1/XX

POLICY

The following is to serve as a guide for orientation of all personnel employed at Anytown Physical Therapy Clinic. Orientation will be provided by the Director of Physical Therapy.

1. Introduction
   (a) Practice hours of operation.
   (b) Work schedule.
   (c) Pay Periods.
   (d) Insurance programs.
   (e) Read job descriptions.
2. Daily Operations
   (a) Tour practice facility.
   (b) Daily patient schedule.
   (c) Modality review.
   (d) Read practice policies and procedures.
3. Safety Program
   (a) Fire evacuation plan.
   (b) Film on body mechanics.
   (c) Emergency procedures.
4. Comments:

Employee Signature _____

Director's Signature _____

Date _____

CHAPTER ELEVEN

MARKETING IN PRIVATE PRACTICE

A S COMPETITION intensifies and health care costs continue to rise an increasing number of physical therapists are investigating the use of marketing in the private practice setting. As many physical therapists soon discover, however, they often lack the professional training and experience to properly apply health care marketing principles to practice operations. Because of this, practitioners often spend thousands of dollars on marketing efforts which provide little, if any, benefit to the practice or serve to stimulate practice growth.

The most common mistake for an individual who is unaccustomed to the use of marketing in health care is to see it as nothing more than public relations. It is natural that marketing's most valuable components, advertising and promotion, are often mistaken as representing the entire field of thought. After all, when a promotional strategy fails, the tendency is to place blame for the failure on the individual promotional effort or the advertising media chosen.

To apply marketing to a private practice requires an understanding of the term by the practitioner. This chapter discusses how the marketing concept in health care can be adapted for use in either a new or established private practice. Because of the characteristics of the physical therapy profession, the task of developing a total marketing program for a private practice can be challenging. The application of marketing to a physical therapy practice can, however, be advantageous to both the patient and the therapist. Marketing can improve the quality of health care offered, and give the practitioner a more competitive edge in providing health care services.

THE MARKETING CONCEPT

In order for marketing to be of benefit to the private practitioner, there must be an adoption of the marketing concept. Simply defined, the marketing concept means that all the practice's efforts are directed towards satisfying patients at a profit.

Understanding the marketing concept will allow the practitioner to better understand and treat patients. The practitioner may also find it is easier to obtain patient compliance and therefore better rehabilitation results. Those practitioners who believe in the marketing concept know that satisfaction of patient needs should be the main focus of the practice.

The marketing concept calls for changing the practice's orientation towards the patient. Viewed from this perspective, marketing is not a cluster of techniques so much as it is an orientation and a process that attempts to systematically plan, study, and manage relationships between patients and the practice.

Health care marketing does not mean advertising, even though that may be one way to reach the perspective patient. Marketing is an attempt to position the practice in a community in such a manner that it fulfills an unsatisfied patient need. It fulfills this need by offering medical services that are either unavailable or only partially available in a community. Marketing can be essential to the success of implementing a new patient service or a treatment technique.

If taken seriously, the health care marketing concept can be a very powerful tool for the private practice. It forces the practice members to (1) think through what is being done and, (2) develop a plan for accomplishing a given set of objectives. Where the marketing concept is accepted and applied, it quite often leads to higher profits and increased productivity.

USES FOR MARKETING IN PRACTICE

There are four ways in which marketing may be utilized by the private practitioner. Each represents unique opportunities and applications depending on the practice situation.

1. Entrenchment

This marketing philosophy is an attempt to "dig in" and retain the patient load already established by the practice. Primarily used for established private practices, it is usually in response to increased competition. This approach can, however, help to build a practice by the generation of a large number of referrals from patients currently treated by the practice.

2. Developing New Services

A marketing philosophy which can be used by either a new or established practitioner. For the new practitioner, it means to establish a practice which offers services unlike any other practitioner in the community. The established practitioner can, on the other hand, add a new dimension to a practice by changing some of the present services or by adding new services.

3. Market Development

A marketing philosophy directed towards making potential patients aware of the practice. Market development can be used by an established or new practice. The primary purpose of market development is to promote only those services presently offered by the practice.

4. Practice Diversification

A practitioner who diversifies is one who moves into a totally different line of business. The most challenging opportunities involve practice diversification. An example of diversification would be a practitioner who owns a small practice and decides to expand into creating a home health agency. Here both new services and new markets are included.

PRACTICE MARKET PLANNING MODEL

To utilize marketing in a practice there must be a development of a marketing plan. A marketing plan is a six-step process which will allow the identification of all potential aspects of a community that could influence practice operations. From the careful evaluation of a community, the practitioner will then be able to develop specific objectives which will allow for the efficient allocation of resources. These resources include the practice's staff, time, equipment, and money.

Practice Market Planning Model

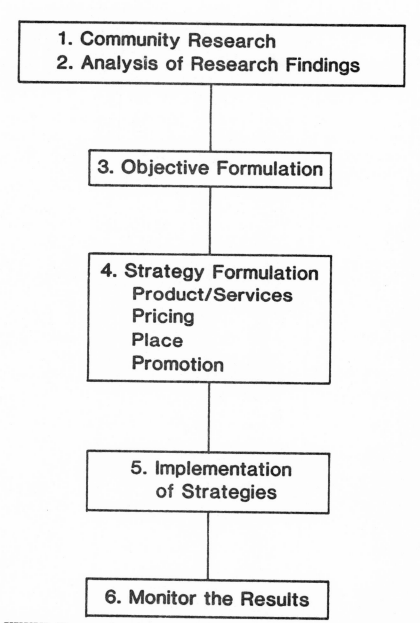

Figure XXXVI. The steps in private practice marketing. Any step can be modified to adjust for changes in the environment of the practitioner.

The essential components of a private practice marketing plan are:

1. Community Research. If the practitioner is astute, research will be as thorough as possible. Research is basic to a complete understanding of patient needs and the relative competition in the community.

2. Analysis of Research Findings. Having collected the research, the next question must be, "How do I use the findings?" Careful review of the findings will tell you a great deal about the community. The research findings should also provide information about the potential success or failure of any proposed marketing effort.

3. Set Practice Objectives. As in any business, you must develop objectives and goals you would like to see accomplished by the practice. These can include a variety of functions including the attraction of a new patient group to the practice.

4. Strategy Formulation. The objective is to formulate the actions necessary to realize objectives and goals. Strategies identify the target market and the marketing mixes needed to attract the desired type of patient.

5. Implementation of the Strategies. Introduction of new services to a patient group means they must be both accessible and available. You must attempt to introduce any new service at both the right place and right time.

6. Monitor the Results. The practitioner must, at all times, monitor the results of any new marketing program. Depending on patient and community response, rapid changes may need to be made to make the marketing effort successful.

DEVELOPING A MARKETING PLAN

Before you can begin to develop a new patient service you must determine how your patients view the practice. To understand the patients, you must at least attempt to recognize their concerns and opinions. The greater the distance between you and your patients, the less chance a marketing program will be successful. The successful development of a marketing plan must therefore begin with community research.

Step One: Community Research

One way to initiate a marketing research program for private practice is by obtaining statistics on the local community from the chamber of commerce or city government. Data supplied by these institutions can help in compiling a profile of the market by age, average income, and family size. There can also be a geographic breakdown of the population which indicates where people are moving from and where they are moving to.

It is also essential to answer the following questions about the community. These questions will profile areas of the population which may not have been investigated by the state or local governments.

Ten Important Questions

1. What is the type of patient you would like to attract to the practice? (The "type of patient" is often referred to as the target market.)

2. What patient needs do you perceive are not being met by other physical therapy practitioners? Could you open a practice or expand an existing one to meet those needs?

3. Considering your professional background and experience, what particular advantage do you offer in patient treatment?

4. What medical specialities will most likely refer you patients on a regular basis?

5. Is the community stable? What is the economic forecast?

6. How many other practitioners will or are competing with you for patients?

7. Do patients have a choice in where they go for physical therapy services?

8. Considering your practice location, is it convenient to a large percentage of patients?

9. What services could the practice offer which would require no additional personnel or increase office expenses?

10. What attitude do the people in the community have towards physical therapy? Are they aware of the services which can be offered by a physical therapist?

Step Two: Analysis of Research Findings

Once research has been conducted, the next important step is to interpret the statistical findings. For example, what information is provided which will help the practitioner make a better decision regarding practice operations? The analysis of research findings is often the most difficult part of health care marketing. The practitioner must make every effort to evaluate the data objectively. It is essential the practitioner avoid interjecting personal biases or opinions which alter the review of data.

Analyzing the Answers to the Ten Questions

The main objective to developing a set of questions for use in analysis of a community, is to obtain data which is of value to the practice. A practitioner may develop any number of questions depending on the type and size of the market to be examined. The ten questions presented will allow the practitioner to analyze the following community related factors.

Question One: This question is designed to provide a starting point for the established practitioner. When undertaking the marketing of any new service, you must decide the patient load or target market. The patient load or target market is a group of patients who often have very similar health care needs. Examples of specific target markets are those consisting of orthopaedic, neurological, and pediatric patients. Each requires different rehabilitative services and techniques.

Question Two: Every practitioner should attempt to identify those areas of patient care not provided in a community. Once identified, the practitioner can then look for ways to offer these services. Often vital community services are not provided which, if offered, would greatly expand a practice.

Question Three: Your professional training, experience, and personal interests are to be determined by this question. It is imperative that you seek out a market opportunity which provides you with professional and personal satisfaction.

Question Four: To properly answer this question means you must attempt to identify the needs of the local medical community. You may have an excellent idea for expansion into a new patient market, but will the medical community support it?

Question Five: Some communities in the United States are in a profound state of economic change. In some northern cities, for example, the steel and automotive industries have suffered larger personnel lay-offs. An idea to market a new service in a depressed community may be excellent, but few individuals may be able to afford it.

Question Six: Your new marketing program may involve the development of a back school. Before starting any new venture, investigate how many local practitioners have a similar project. Are their endeavors financially successful?

Question Seven: A large percentage of patients with a specific type of disability may be accustomed to receiving therapy at one designated facility. What services can you offer which will attract some of these patients to your practice?

Question Eight: Are you conveniently located for the market which you would like to attract? The facility should be easily accessible or patients will probably go to a more convenient location.

Question Nine: Involvement in community-related activities will increase the publics' awareness of the practice. Advertising can be very expensive and should be avoided unless it will provide wide exposure to a specific target market.

Question Ten: Assess the community's awareness of the physical therapy profession. You may find there is a need to inform the public how important it is that they utilize physical therapy prior to starting a new marketing program.

Step Three: Objective Formulation

Once there has been a determination of an area of practice you would like to change, improve, or expand, the next step is to set objectives for its accomplishment. The answers to the ten questions will be the basis for carrying out the process of setting practice objectives. When formulating objectives or goals, it is important that each one be specific so that its progress or lack of progress can be assessed. The following case illustrates to process of objective formulation.

The Case: Developing a Sports Medicine Program

A private practitioner researched a community and determined the local high school was quite active in sporting events but had been unable to locate an individual to provide athletic training and emergency assistance at home games. The school originally approached an orthopaedic surgeon to provide assistance, but quite frequently, surgical emergencies limited his attendance.

The practitioner had extensive training, interest, and education in the field of sports medicine. The practitioner decided to pursue the opportunity to become involved in sports medicine at the community level. It was determined that most of the involvement was to be in the early evenings. This time was very convenient since it would allow the practitioner to continue normal practice operations and also provide the opportunity to expand the practice's area of expertise.

The practitioner therefore set the objective as: Increase the practices' present sports medicine patient volume by 15 percent within one year.

Goals such as these are reasonable and easy to assess. This goal provides a quantitative means to assess the changes in patient volume. The goal also specifies a time frame in which to be accomplished. The one-year goal will allow the practitioner to become involved in all sporting activities at the high school level.

Step Four:
Strategy Formulation and the Marketing Mixes

After the formulation of objectives, the practitioner must devise a plan (strategy) by which each objective can be accomplished. Marketing strategies are essential to properly identify the target market and the marketing mix.

In health care marketing, the target market and the marketing mix are defined as follows:

1. Target Market. A similar group of patients to whom the practice would like to appeal.

2. Marketing Mix. The controllable group of variables the practitioner puts together in order to satisfy the needs of the target market.

It is important to recognize that a marketing strategy will focus on some particular target patient. The reason to focus on a specific target patient is to gain a competitive advantage. The competitive advantage is gained through a greater understanding of patients with similar needs and rehabilitation requirements.

In the case presented, the practitioner decided to start the sports medicine program with a target market of the high school boy's soccer team. The practitioner believed this would be an excellent way to introduce the endurance, flexibility, and training concepts of sports medicine physical therapy in an essentially noncontact sport. Since the incidence of injury is low in soccer, compared to contact sports, the practitioner hoped to be able to introduce the physical therapy profession in a more preventative medicine approach.

DEVELOPING PATIENT MARKETING MIXES

There are a number of ways to satisfy the needs of the target market. The best way to reduce the number of potential variables which must be considered is to group them into four areas. Each require special consideration when applied to health care marketing in a private practice These areas are:

Product/Service
Place
Promotion
Price

Product/Service

Medical care is for the most part not considered a product, but a service. A product is something which is tangible. A service is an activity that a private practitioner can offer to a patient which does not result in ownership of anything which is tangible.

No matter how it is viewed, you direct all your efforts to assist the patients in their rehabilitation. Your entire "product" consists of your education, experiences, professional opinions, and the skill and treatment methods by which you practice physical therapy.

In the case presented, the service provided will consist of the practitioners' specialized knowledge and abilities in the area of athletic injuries, physical conditioning, and rehabilitation. The practitioner will attempt to offer these services to decrease the chance of injury and increase athletic performance.

Place

The primary concern in any health care marketing effort is to get the service to the target market. Depending on the selection of a target market, the location the service is to be offered will vary. A service, such as physical therapy, isn't much good to a patient if it isn't available when and where it is needed.

In the sports medicine example, the service would primarily be offered on the field of play. The practitioner would be expected to volunteer time to the high school's athletic activities. Through repeated exposure, the practitioner hopes to see the practice recognized as a community leader in rehabilitation. When an injury needs to be rehabilitated, it is hoped the athlete will choose the practitioner's facility.

Promotion

A good channel of communication is essential to properly promote a private practice. The target market must know the physical therapy services are available and how they can best be acquired. Personal selling is often a very effective means of promoting a practice.

Personal selling involves direct, face-to-face communication between the practitioner and the potential patients. It is essential that potential patients become aware of the practice's services so they automatically think of you when it comes time to seek rehabilitation.

Besides personal selling, a practitioner can also communicate effectively through advertising. To advertise frequently means you must pay to get the message across. Many practitioners utilize one or more of the following to advertise the practice: (1) newspapers, (2) business cards, (3) yellow pages, or (4) printed announcements.

Before selecting an advertising program, determine who will be the primary target market. For example, relaying technical treatment information to a group of medical doctors may require a different advertising program than would be required to inform potential patients of the services offered by the practice.

Price

Patients realize the time and treatments provided by the practice require payment. Many of the services you must provide to attract a target market cannot, however, be compensated. A new practitioner will spend countless hours in community service projects which provide little or no monetary rewards. Quite often, it takes this to develop a practice.

When setting a price for health care services, the practitioner must consider the competition present in the community. To develop a new marketing program, the practitioner must be realistic about all charges for patient treatment. The compassion you demonstrate in patient charges and in the collection of fees is part of personal selling.

Step Five: Implementation of Strategies

As a marketing strategy is implemented, it must be done with the thought in mind that it may need to be altered depending on patient response. The implementation of strategy can be a gradual process or a rapid event. Quite often, competition determines how quickly a strategy must be implemented.

In the case presented, the practitioner chose to gradually implement a one-year strategy to provide health care services to a local high school. This is a planned process whereby each sporting activity will be offered athletic training and rehabilitative services.

If the community were competitive, the practitioner may have to seek a more rapid implementation. When several health care practitioners are attempting to provide services, the one with the best marketing strategy quite often will come out on top.

Step Six: Monitoring the Results

The final step in a marketing plan for a private practice is an ongoing one. The results of your efforts must continually be measured to see if the practice is reaching its desired objectives and goals.

A marketing strategy, even if successful, must be updated. Patient attitudes and rehabilitation needs quite often change with time. The practitioner who does not monitor the marketing results will often soon discover patient volume is decreasing. Patient volume often decreases because someone else found a better way to market and provide rehabilitative services. To be successful, the practitioner must continually direct efforts towards letting the target market know where to obtain the latest in specialized health care services.

KEEP THE STAFF INVOLVED

There are two ingredients which will keep patients satisfied. One is the practitioner's rapport with the patient. The other is the attitude of staff members. Your professional and economic success will depend on the professionalism and dedication staff members have towards the practice's health care marketing program.

Consumer orientation, the process of thinking in terms of patient needs and wants, must be the primary direction of the practice and its staff members. To obtain the cooperation of staff members in any marketing effort, thoroughly explain what attempts you are making to expand or change current practice operations. All staff members must be aware of the image the practice is attempting to portray. The final outcome of any marketing program is often contingent upon the staff's support in portraying that practice image.

CHAPTER TWELVE

COMPUTERS IN PRIVATE PRACTICE

D URING THE past five years, the computer has emerged on the medical practice scene. This small, relatively inexpensive machine can greatly improve the overall operating efficiency of a private practice. The computer can store large amounts of information in a small space with greater speed, flexibility, and accuracy than a manual system.

A computerized practice offers three important advantages to the practitioner. One commonly cited advantage is the speed of computer calculations. Todays' computer can make vital practice calculations several times faster than can be performed by hand. When attached to a printer, the practitioner can obtain financial results in only a few short minutes. These results can be obtained whenever needed with little manual effort.

A second advantage to computerization in private practice is the accuracy of the information provided. There are a number of programs, for example, which instantly provide information on the age of a patient's account, or the diagnosis profile by the physician. As long as the data is entered correctly, the computer output results will be accurate.

The third advantage to computerization is the information storage capacity. Modern computer manufacturers have developed machines which have large memories. In most cases, almost all patient record information can be stored on one machine. Once stored, this eliminates the necessity of reentering information each time a calculation must be made.

COMPUTER TERMINOLOGY

In order to understand the many functions that a computer can perform, the practitioner must first become familiar with some of the

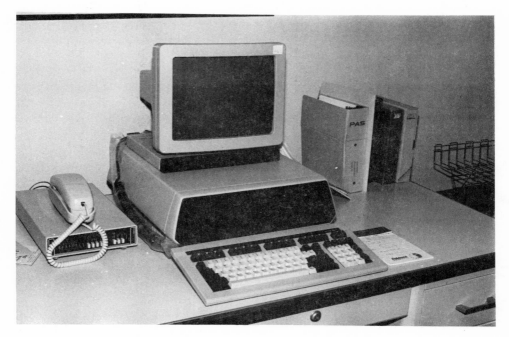

Figure XXXVII. Private practice computer with keyboard and video screen.

terminology common to the computer industry. It is not necessary to become a computer expert in order to utilize a machine in practice. It will, however, be of invaluable assistance to already be familiar with basic computer terminology when discussing computer applications with a salesperson.

To begin with, the practitioner must be aware of the differences between computer hardware and computer software. Hardware refers to the microcomputer. There are several types of computers. The ones which sit on desk tops and contain small micro chips are called microcomputers. This is the computer most utilized by health care providers.

Hardware also includes the printer, and other physical equipment such as the keyboard, needed to operate the machine. The video screen, frequently seen placed on top of the computer, is also considered part of the computer hardware.

Computer software refers to the programs necessary to operate the machine. The software provides a set of instructions which allows the computer hardware to perform desired functions. Software is generally stored on a diskette or "floppy disk." The diskette looks like a small phonograph record encased in a protective cover. The protective cover prevents damage during repeated handling.

Many computers and software systems for use in a medical practice are designed to be user-friendly. User-friendly is a term used to describe the computer and software package which are developed to meet the needs of the beginner. This is not to say, however, that they will not perform complex practice functions. They are simply designed to be easy to use.

COMPUTER APPLICATIONS IN PRACTICE

There are a number of functions that a microcomputer can perform for a private practice. Most of these functions will lead to increased practice productivity and efficiency. They provide benefits to the practice by better controlling operations and reducing costs.

In health care, there are two distinct areas in which a microcomputer will be of benefit. These areas are for financial analysis of the practice and for word processing. Many software programs have been written for these two areas. The following section examines these two types of software in more detail.

The Financial Aspects

Software most commonly available to assist in the financial aspects of practice include those programs for preparation of the practice payroll, general ledger, accounts payable, and accounts receivable. Each provides valuable financial assistance to the practitioner.

The Practice Payroll

Having the practice payroll on computer can reduce the time consuming process of maintaining hand prepared payroll records. Payroll checks can be computer generated along with reports concerning Social Security (F.I.C.A.) as well as state and federal withholding tax.

There may also be a record of employee contributions to benefit and pension programs. When needed, the computer can update an employee's salary record for a given pay period or for the calendar year. The computer can also be used to record unpaid leaves of absence and loans made to employees. These records may be reviewed on a weekly, monthly, quarterly, or annual basis. At years end, the computer may also be used to generate tax reports and W-2 forms.

The General Ledger

A general ledger program can be very valuable to a practice. Software packages such as these can prepare income statements, balance sheets, and itemize office expenses. The general ledger program will allow the practitioner to determine the financial position of the practice at any time.

In some practice situations, the general ledger program can virtually replace the need for a full-time bookkeeper. The computer cannot, however, replace the need for a practice accountant. The accountant will always be needed to provide financial information on changes in tax laws. The practice accountant should also periodically review all data generated by the computer. This will ensure information is being correctly entered into the computer.

Accounts Receivable

One of the most popular programs is accounts receivable. This program provides information about how much money is owed to the practice by patients. In general, the longer a patient goes without paying their bill, the more money it costs the practice. The older the patient account, the less likely you are to collect for your services.

The accounts receivable program can be used to improve collection efficiency. The system is designed to provide information as to how long an account has been outstanding. Depending on the software system, the computer may be able to generate standardized collection letters. Collection letters should begin as gentle reminders for payment and then proceed to a more demanding request.

The Accounts Payable Program

The accounts payable program will provide information about what bills the practice needs to pay. For example, when a bill arrives it can be entered into the computer as an amount that needs to be payed. When additional billing statements arrive, the computer can check the present billing statement against information already on file concerning the amount owed.

The accounts payable program will help avoid many problems with accounts becoming overdue or lost in the mail. Once it is determined the practice is liable for the bill, some programs will allow the computer to issue a check for the correct amount.

WORD PROCESSING PROGRAMS

One of the most popular nonfinancial uses to computerization in private practice is for word processing. A word processing software program will allow the practitioner to create, edit, retrieve, and print material without the time-consuming process of typing or retyping letters.

In the past, errors on letters and documents frequently meant retyping. With word processing, the typist simply backs up and types over the error. Changes can be made to documents without retyping the entire document. Once completed, the document can be printed in final form.

Word processing reduces the need for a copy machine since information can be kept in the computer or on a floppy diskette. This helps to reduce filing costs and allows more time to perform patient-related activities.

An important feature of a word processing program is the ability for information entered to "wrap." The wrap feature (sometimes called "wrap around") means the typist does not have to strike the return key at the end of each line. The program will automatically move the sentence to the next line. This will allow information to be entered quickly with little or no hesitation.

Another important feature of word processing is the ability of the program to provide personal correspondence. This feature allows you to personalize letters by extracting information from a list of records. When it is time to mail letters, you simply instruct the program to print a personalized letter to each recipient.

OTHER USES FOR WORD PROCESSING

1. Referral letters.
2. Thank you letters.
3. Collection letters.
4. Letters to patients (appointment changes, acknowledgement of payments received).
5. Letters to physicians (announcing a new treatment method, information requests, invitations to presentations).
6. Letters to fellow professionals.
7. Letters to professional associations.
8. Letters for order placement.
9. Requests for information.

Will word processing be beneficial to your practice? Consider how frequently you use these standardized documents. The more identical the documents, the greater the value of word processing.

COMPUTERS AND INSURANCE

Completing an insurance claim form for a patient is a time-consuming task. Some practitioners have tried to reduce the volume of paperwork by simply refusing to accept the burden of filing a patient's insurance. Patients do, however, also find the process of filing their own insurance claims annoying. As competition in the health care industry continues to increase, the practitioner who offers to process a patient's insurance claim may be helping to build the practice.

In most practice situations insurance forms are received on a daily basis. There are, however, very few practices who have enough office personnel to complete the forms on a daily basis. A good insurance claim processing system requires constant employee effort for maximum results.

Depending on the computer software chosen for the practice, it may be possible to submit insurance claims directly from the office computer to the insurance company's computer. This can be done via the telephone lines. If your practice has a large volume of claims to be filed with one insurance carrier, such as medicare, it is essential you investigate which type of insurance hardware and software that will be needed. This "paperless" claims processing will not only reduce the number of phone calls from patients concerning their insurance but will also decrease the likelihood of undetected errors, reduced payment allowances, and delays in claims processing.

THE COST-BENEFIT ANALYSIS

One aspect which must be investigated before making the decision to purchase a computer is the relative cost-benefit analysis. A cost-benefit analysis means that every computer system must be cost-justified. The computer must pay for itself and make a financial contribution to the practice.

There are some practice functions that are best performed manually. That is because it would simply be too expensive to computerize them.

In other cases the software may be available but at too costly of a price. The practitioner must, therefore, investigate the costs associated with maintaining current operations as opposed to computerization.

There are three areas to carefully examine when performing a cost-benefit analysis. They are productivity, expenses, and collections.

Productivity

A private practice can show a definite increase in productivity through computerization. Once employees fully understand how to use the computer, information can be processed much faster. This will provide the employee with more time to spend with patients. In some instances, computerization will allow the practice to see more patients while maintaining the same level of high quality patient care.

One way to assess the value of a computer is to analyze the current productivity of the staff. There are five areas which should be assessed prior to making the investment decision. They are: (1) is there a long delay in processing insurance forms? (2) Is the staff spending more time with paperwork and less time treating patients? (3) Is information lacking about the diagnosis most often treated, the most frequently used modality, and the physician referring the greatest number of patients? (4) how many hours per week are spent on office functions which could be computerized? (5) what is the total number of active patients? Is the practice growing?

Also evaluate how hard the staff is working. The best time to evaluate this is when you are considering hiring another person to perform typing or insurance work. In many cases, the addition of a computer can lessen the need for additional personnel.

Expenses

If you are paying individuals overtime to complete insurance forms that translates into lost practice income. Over a period of several years, a computer could more than pay for itself. A practice grossing $150,000 might well have expenses of $60,000 to $70,000 or more. If you could reduce expenses by five percent you could easily save the practice $3,000 to $3,500 yearly.

Collections

If the computer can be used to closely keep track of over-due accounts, it can potentially increase practice income. Assume it currently takes, on average, three to four months to fully collect on a patient's account. Suppose, however, you were able to reduce that period of time by one month. That would greatly enhance the financial performance of the practice.

CHOOSE THE SOFTWARE, THEN THE HARDWARE

The most important part of computerizing a private practice is the proper selection of the software. Software selection will often dictate the type of hardware chosen.

The software is what will provide the operating instructions to the computer hardware. What functions you want performed by the software will influence hardware requirements. The most common applications for computers in medical offices are for: (1) practice accounting, (2) patient billing, (3) insurance claims, (4) accounts payable, (5) practice payroll, (6) appointment scheduling, (7) general ledger, (8) word processing, (9) medical records, (10) telecommunications.

User-friendly software packages frequently require more computer memory. Adjustments may also need to be made based on the type of printer required to perform the necessary functions. As a general rule, once the software decisions are made, the choice of hardware is much easier.

THE CHOICE OF HARDWARE

The first choice of hardware should always be the central processing unit or C.P.U. There are some important areas to investigate prior to purchase. They are as follows:

1. What are the computer's limitations? The practitioner must assess the limitations of the computer's memory. Small computers have only 64,000 bytes of memory (sometimes called 64K). The important question is whether or not the computer can be expanded or "upgraded" to provide a greater memory as the practice grows.

2. How many terminals can the computer accommodate at the same time? Can it be expanded? Can all the terminals be used at the same time? One of the most important features to a growing practice is the ability of the computer to execute two or more programs at the same time. Can one employee perform word processing while another enters

data on a new patient? Some computer systems can perform only one function at a time. Other computers will allow several employees to enter and retrieve data simultaneously. Do not let the limitations of the computer hinder office efficiency.

NEGOTIATING THE BEST PRICE

When the practitioner has decided that a microcomputer would be an asset to the practice, the next step is to purchase the machine. To purchase a computer often requires some negotiation. This is because, regardless of price, many retailers will often make price concessions on computer software and hardware. Depending on the retailer, you may be able to obtain as much as 5 to 10 percent off the list price.

Many retailers also sell service contracts on all computer hardware. The price for a service contract frequently runs 10 percent of the total price of the hardware. An annual service contract on a six thousand dollar computer will be approximately six hundred dollars for the first year.

It may be advisable to purchase a service contract. If there is a major problem with a six thousand dollar computer, it will likely cost in excess of six hundred dollars to correct. Some service contracts can be successfully negotiated downward. Once again, however, have a clear understanding of what services are covered before purchasing the service agreement.

THE COMPUTER INSTALLATION

A computer should be installed in the proper environment in order to provide the best service to the practice. In general, if the office is comfortable for the practice employees and patients, it probably will be comfortable enough for the computer. There are, however, some recommendations for the best environment for both the computer and the employees who will be working with the machine.

TEMPERATURE CONTROL

Temperatures for most computers and computer equipment should be between fifty and ninety degrees fahrenheit with relatively low humidity. High humidity may cause condensation which could damage internal computer components. It is therefore advisable for humidity levels to range from forty to no higher than eighty percent.

To adequately protect computer equipment from high humidity, do not install any computer components near whirlpool areas. Purchase a humidity gauge and periodically check the area surrounding the computer. On weekends, set the air conditioner levels at eighty degrees. This will protect the equipment without causing high practice electric bills.

POWER SOURCE PROTECTION

A fluctuation in power supply to the computer can cause damage to the internal components. To protect against damage, install a surge protector. All computer equipment, including the printer should be plugged into a surge protector. In stormy weather, do not operate any computer equipment. Instead, unplug all computer related equipment.

LOCATION OF THE COMPUTER

Many of today's private practices were not designed with the intent to implement the computer into practice operation. It is therefore sometimes difficult to find a place to set up the computer. For many practitioners, the most desirable location for the computer is at or near the receptionist's desk. This will allow the receptionist to perform the daily practice operations while entering data into the machine at the same time.

The computer should never be placed in direct sunlight since this may cause overheating. Adequate ventilation is a must while the machine is in operation. When not in use, the machine should be covered with a dust cover.

TELEPHONE LINES

In order to transmit computer insurance information to an insurance company, the computer will need a device called a modem. The modem converts data entered into the computer into a form compatible with transmission through telephone lines.

Insurance claims can be processed quickly through the use of telephone lines if your machine is properly equiped. To avoid interference and interruption in transmission, the computer company may recommend a separate telephone line to transmit computer messages and information.

OPERATOR COMFORT

When installing a computer, give careful consideration to the physical characteristics of the person primarily responsible for entering the data. The proper height for both the keyboard and the monitor is essential. Setting the keyboard height at twenty-six to twenty-eight inches above the floor should provide the most convenience. Monitor height should be slightly higher but no higher than eye level.

A comfortable chair should be provided which gives adequate support to the low back and legs. The operator should always face the computer and be provided with enough desk top space for all required work. If the computer operator is required to work for long periods while entering data, encourage frequent breaks. This helps reduce eye strain and muscle fatigue.

INSTALLATION

The actual job of setting up the computer should be the responsibility of one of the computer company's technical staff. Each component of the computer should be tested to ensure its proper operation. No equipment should be accepted which appears to have been damaged or used as a demonstrator model.

Once the computer has been properly set up, the software will be installed. The first software to be installed will be the operating system software. The operating system software enables each component of hardware to work together to properly execute the application software.

The installation of the application software will follow after a series of diagnostic tests are performed to ensure the computer is functioning properly. The application software will include the medical management package. The medical management package will be used in the daily operations of the practice.

COMPUTER TRAINING THE STAFF

The final step in computer installation is making the system work to increase practice operations and efficiency. The success of any computer system in private practice largely depends on the employees who will operate it. Because of this, a number of problems can develop.

One problem that frequently develops is the threat the employees feel towards job security. To those employees who have never used a computer, the mere thought of being forced to use one can be a source of great anxiety. Frequently, they fear their old job will be replaced by the operations of the computer. In some cases, they may express anxiety over possible failure that may result in their dismissal. These sources of anxiety are often a reaction to the resistance to change.

No matter the source of anxiety, it must be addressed. It is important that the staff be reassured and provided with proper training to become proficient in the use of the computer. It should be explained to each employee that additional tasks will be found to replace the ones which were computerized.

Another common problem is employee resistance to the utilization of information provided by the computer. Since the computer will provide rapid up-to-date information, the practice personnel will be expected to act upon the data provided. Computer systems will provide up-to-date information on accounts which have become overdue. The practice personnel will be expected to contact overdue patient accounts by letter or phone for prompt payment. The easiest way to handle problems such as these is to explain the value to the practice of these services. Through careful and thorough explanations, the practitioner can gain their assistance and cooperation.

An additional problem is that, at least in the initial stages, the greatest amount of attention will be focused on solving problems. Many of these problems can be avoided, or at least minimized, by a computer company who provides a formal training session. A company which is committed to the success of its computer system will provide several days of training for a medical management software system. Additional time may be needed if the software is extremely complex.

All computer training of employees should be conducted by an individual who is proficient in the operation of the system, recognizes employee inexperience, and knows how private practices work. Some companies will provide a computer hot line for periods up to one year to answer questions and diagnose computer problems. Ask the representative about the training to be provided. Inquire as to how much assistance will be provided to get the system operating and keep it going the first six months to one year.

Every individual in the practice who will be responsible for operating the computer should receive formal training. Some companies will train only one operator who is then expected to train others in the practice. This can create a multiple of problems. The employees should be trained as a group so they can work to solve problems in a group fashion. The company who tries to teach just one person is cutting corners and should be avoided.

Training sessions almost always involve the entire staff for a full day. During the days of formal training, it is best if patient treatment is kept to a minimum. Employees should not be distracted with the daily operations of the practice. In areas where employees have difficulty retaining important information, record the company representative's presentation on cassette tape.

Company presented training sessions should take the employee through all rudimentary computer functions. A presentation should include instruction on practice functions such as creating a computer record for a patient, posting charges, and aging individual accounts receivable. Inexperienced operators should practice newly acquired skills on sample data. This data should approximate the actual data which will be processed by the computer system.

FURTHER PRACTICE ANALYSIS

It is important to assess the growth of the practice. A computer system in a private practice will not help the business grow. It will, however, increase the stream of revenue as growth begins to occur. To provide maximum benefit, the computer system should help save the practice money and increase operating efficiency.

Computer system quality will vary. It is important to shop around for both computer hardware and software. If you purchase a computer of poor quality or encounter a dealer with a poor service department, you could loose several thousand dollars.

The best way to assess your needs is to become familiar with the computer industry and what it has to offer. The following are examples of individuals or groups who should be consulted prior to purchase.

1. Talk with fellow professionals. Begin by consulting fellow practitioners about the systems they have installed in their office. Most of these suggestions will involve changes they would make "if they could do it again."

2. Read computer literature. Find out as much as you can about computer systems for small business. Consult the local library or college about classes in computers and word processing.

3. Attend computer shows. Almost every major city has at least one computer show. The computer show is often sponsored by several major manufacturers of computers in cooperation with local computer retailers. These shows will allow the practitioner to compare several computer systems under one roof.

4. Computer clubs. These clubs are formed by individuals who have a great deal of interest in computers and computer software. Members of these clubs work together in solving hardware problems and exchanging computer software. Many times, individual club members can provide invaluable assistance in the selection and set-up of a computer system. Consult the local library for meeting times and location.

IF NECESSARY, CONSULT A PROFESSIONAL

Whether or not you need a computer is a decision that can only be made after careful analysis of the practice. The review of the office business practices can be done by you and your fellow employees. If necessary, there are also professionals, such as management consultants, who can evaluate practice efficiency and offer suggestions.

No matter who does the evaluation, it is essential that the study investigate practice productivity. Increasing efficiency and productivity translates into larger gross income. Implementing a computer system in an office can be difficult. Patient care encompasses not only treatment but also office management. The physical therapist who is both efficient and organized will have a more satisfied group of patients and employees.

CHAPTER THIRTEEN

SUCCESSFUL MANAGERS
AND TIMETABLES FOR PRACTICE

TO OPEN a private practice takes a considerable amount of planning and risk taking. No small business, especially a medical practice, is risk free. There is always a chance you will improperly analyze the environment and suffer a financial loss.

Environmental analysis is, however, only part of what it takes to go into private practice. There are certain managerial traits which appear to influence entrepreneural success. This chapter investigates those traits as well as presenting a timetable to assist in opening a new practice. Every prospective practitioner must be aware of the traits of successful managers and some of the many tasks which must be performed prior to opening an office. A physical therapist should not consider opening a new practice without establishing a target date.

CHARACTERISTICS WHICH CONTRIBUTE
TOWARD SUCCESS IN MANAGERIAL POSITIONS

Those in business have long searched to identify the personality characteristics that contribute to business success. Unfortunately, there has been no firm agreement as to what makes the best business leader. It is clear, however, some individuals are better suited to be employees, while others would much rather be employers.

The private practitioner is in every way an entrepreneur. The owner of the practice organizes all aspects of the business and takes responsibility for its success or failure. There is no complete list of traits or characteristics to describe every business person. There are, however, some that tend to be common in many successful business people. They are: technical knowledge, mental ability, human relations skills, drive to achieve, and creativity. Each of these warrant close attention.

Technical Knowledge

One of the most important characteristics in small business is for the practitioner to know what he or she is doing. In order to open a private practice you must be well versed in all aspects of the profession, the treatment of patients, and in the technical aspects of medicine. Technical knowledge is one ability that a physical therapist can acquire with effort. If you are interested in private practice, you must be the type of individual who is well acquainted with the profession and the wide variety of services it has to offer.

Mental Ability

The private practitioner must be one who can recognize problems and develop ways of solving them. Those individuals who are best in small business situations are generalists. A generalist is a person who can look at the practice in broad terms and develop strategies to change the direction of a practice or to solve problems. To be successful, the practitioner must be reasonably intelligent, able to adapt managerial actions to the needs of the practice, and know how jobs interrelate.

Human Relations Skills

Personality factors such as socialability, consideration, communication ability, and tactfulness are all important aspects of human relations skills. The practitioner must be able to put his or herself "in another's position" before taking any action. The practitioner should be skilled in establishing relations with patients, employees, and the medical community. To do this requires effective communication. Effective communication can be achieved by following a series of basic communication principles.

1. Always think before communicating.
2. Use face to face communication whenever possible.
3. Try to communicate in a way that is helpful to the person receiving the message.

4. Give the person a chance to ask questions about what has been communicated.

5. Remember words have different meanings to different people. Make sure the person understands what is communicated to them.

Drive to Achieve

The drive to achieve is a person's motivation toward task accomplishment. People with a high drive to achieve take the personal responsibility for finding the solution to a problem. These same individuals want to take part in the determination of an outcome. They do not want a solution to develop by chance. People with a high drive to achieve want concrete feedback on their performance. In business settings, these people want to know how well they are doing and if it can be improved. These same business people are continually looking for ways to improve the daily business operations. They often make the important business decisions and delegate minor decisions to others.

Creativity

Creativity is the ability of the individual to process information so that the result will either be new or meaningful. Those who are creative are not necessarily brilliant. They simply have a positive image of themselves and like who they are. Creative individuals are challenged by a problem and make a decision only when they believe they have obtained sufficient information. The successful business person who is creative is more concerned with the meaning of the problem than with the finite details.

A TIMETABLE FOR OPENING A PRACTICE

While there are many ways to describe a successful small business owner, one of the most common is organized. To be organized is to develop a plan for use in starting a private practice. The major advantage of a plan is that it forces the practitioner to answer the questions; "Where should I start?", "What problems will I encounter?", and "How will I deal with them?"

A plan for starting a private practice helps to prepare the individual about the conditions he or she may face. The following is a timetable for opening a private practice. It is intended to be used only as a guide. The specific order and recommended dates of completion may change as you get closer to opening your own private practice.

ONE YEAR OR MORE BEFORE OPENING

Indicate When Completed	**Objective**
1. _____	Establish a date for opening the practice.
2.	Investigate where you would like to locate the practice
_____	Check your local library. Each community library can provide information on regions of the country where you might like to establish a practice. Many community libraries maintain a section containing phone books from around the country. Investigate the number of practitioners in a community of interest.
_____	Contact the chamber of commerce in all prospective communities. Ask for population data and community growth information.
_____	Inquire about the local community hospital. What is the bed capacity? Is the occupancy rate high? Does it have plans for expansion? Are physical therapy services widely utilized?
3. _____	Join the Private Practice Section of the American Physical Therapy Association. Talk with members about what areas of the country are best to establish practices.
4. _____	Practice community assessment. Visit several proposed communities and evaluate the practice opportunities.
5. _____	Contact several practitioners in a proposed community. Ask to see their facilities.
6. _____	Write the state licensing board regarding the procedures to obtain physical therapy licensure.
7. _____	Determine where you would like to locate the practice.

NINE MONTHS TO ONE YEAR BEFORE OPENING

1. _____	Determine your personal financial situation. Estimate how much it would cost to start the practice of your interest.

Indicate When Completed	Objective

2. _____ Visit several lending institutions. Talk with the loan officer about what is needed to obtain a loan. Ask for application blanks.

3. _____ Submit loan application forms. Prepare a financial statement showing the projected practice opening date.

4. _____ Investigate several facilities for leasing or purchase.

5. _____ Begin finalizing office layout, design, and physical therapy equipment needs.

6. _____ Contact local city governments about the zoning of the proposed locations. Ask about any anticipated changes.

7. Begin to choose practice consultants:

_____ Accountant (C.P.A.)

_____ Insurance Agent

_____ Real Estate Agent

_____ Attorney

SIX MONTHS BEFORE OPENING

1. Determine office equipment needs:

_____ Calculator/Adding Machine

_____ Photocopy machine

_____ Typewriter

_____ Computer/Word processor

2. _____ Have practice name and phone number printed in the next available listing of the phone book.

3. Investigate opening the following accounts:

_____ Business checking account

_____ Business savings account

_____ Personal checking account

_____ Personal savings account

4. _____ Choose a practice facility.

5. _____ Develop practice budget for first year of operation.

6. _____ If starting a partnership, formulate the agreement and have it signed.

Indicate When Completed	Objective

7.   Determine insurance requirements:
_____ Workers compensation
_____ Auto liability
_____ Property insurance
_____ Disability
_____ Medical
_____ Life
_____ Professional liability
8. _____ Decide on a retirement plan.
9. _____ Obtain provider numbers and procedure coding books.

FOUR MONTHS BEFORE OPENING

1. _____ Design and order sign for the office.
2.   Develop a marketing strategy. Determine:
_____ Product/Service
_____ Promotion
_____ Places
_____ Price
3. _____ Contact the local newspaper for prices of practice announcements.
4. _____ Join local civic organizations.
5. _____ Contact local physicians. Discuss your plans, request they offer suggestions.
6. _____ Talk with local nursing homes and home health agencies about providing physical therapy services.
7. _____ Develop job descriptions for employees.
8. _____ Formulate a private practice policy manual.

THREE MONTHS BEFORE OPENING

1. _____ Develop and order the appointment scheduling book.
2. _____ Begin preliminary interviewing for office assistants and clerical personnel.

Indicate When Completed	Objective

3. _____ Discuss private practice tax requirements with the accountant.

4.   Establish support services:
   _____ Laundry service
   _____ Janitorial service
   _____ Landscaping service

5. _____ Locate a collection agency.

ONE TO TWO MONTHS BEFORE OPENING

1. _____ Establish office hours based on the marketing strategy previously developed.

2.   Order to obtain the following items:
   _____ Appointment cards
   _____ Business cards
   _____ Charge tickets
   _____ Federal and state estimated income forms
   _____ Establish fee schedules
   _____ Locking fire-proof cabinet
   _____ Patient folders
   _____ Charting paper
   _____ Index cards
   _____ Ledger cards
   _____ Stationary and envelopes
   _____ Medical and english dictionary
   _____ Order equipment (medical)
   _____ Purchase drapes, linen, towels, and whirlpool supplies
   _____ Occupational license
   _____ Payroll book
   _____ Fire evacuation plan
   _____ Petty cash box
   _____ Standard insurance forms
   _____ Billing and return envelopes
   _____ Book shelves
   _____ Daysheet and peg-board
   _____ Patient information booklet
   _____ Obtain post office box

Indicate When Completed	Objective
3. _____	Order magazines for reception room
4. _____	Arrange for delivery date of office furniture and medical equipment.

DURING THE LAST MONTH

1. _____	Begin setting up the practice.
2. _____	Turn on utilities.
3. _____	Hire and train the office personnel.
4. _____	Announce an Open House.
5. _____	Contact all possible referral sources in person.
6. _____	Establish a petty cash and change fund.
7. _____	Begin promotional aspects of marketing strategy.
8. _____	Begin scheduling patient appointments.

THE FIRST DAY OF PRACTICE

1. _____	Evaluate and treat the first patient.
2. _____	Reflect on all that has been accomplished. Be proud; You are now a private practice physical therapist!!

FOR THE NEXT SIX MONTHS

The decision to enter private practice should be made with a complete understanding of the risks involved and the ways these risks can be minimized. Establishing a private practice can be a hard competitive struggle. The mortality rate is particularly high for new businesses during the first year of operation.

Why do some businesses fail? In many cases, small businesses fail due to ineffective management. Many businesses should not have been started because the owner lacked managerial "know how," training, and experience. Rather than recognize their weakness, most blame the failure on poor location or excessive competition.

The first six months after opening a new practice are crucial. The practitioner must be attuned to not only the patient's needs but to their own personal style of management. The "competition" will react to your practice with their own marketing plan. You must be prepared to quickly switch directions in order to establish the practice and become a leader in the community.

Many private practitioners are able to realize considerable satisfaction from their work. The challenge of creating a practice and watching it grow can be very exhilarating. Physical therapy is not a business but there is a business side to a private practice in physical therapy. Good business management is essential to providing quality health care services and continued profitability.

GLOSSARY

Abandonment: The withdrawal from the therapist/patient relationship at a crucial point without the patient's consent and without reasonable notice.

Accounts Payable: A current liability incurred when goods or services are purchased on credit.

Accounts Receivable: Claims the practice has against patients for unpaid balances from the performance of services.

Accrual Basis: An accounting term whereby revenue is recognized and reported when it is earned rather than when the resulting cash is collected.

Accumulated Depreciation: The sum of all depreciation charges since the asset was acquired.

Aggregate: A malpractice insurance term describing the total amount which will be paid on any claim.

Aging Accounts Receivable: The process of classifying individual patient accounts by the time which has passed since medical services were rendered.

Allowance for Uncollectables: Those accounts receivable that are judged to be uncollectable.

Amortization: The process of systematically reducing the principle amount of a loan in installments.

Assets: Something of value owned by the practice.

Balance Sheet: A financial statement which reports a practices' financial position at a specific point in time.

Block Scheduling: A method of patient scheduling where each hour is considered a block. Patients are told to come in for treatment on a first-come, first-serve basis.

Break-Even Analysis: A technique for analyzing the relationships among fixed costs, variable costs, and profit.

Budget: A plan with the anticipated results expressed in numerical terms.

Cash: Bank accounts, checks, and currency.

Cash Basis: Income measured on the basis of cash revenues received less cash expenditures.

Cash Surrender Value: A whole life insurance policy which may be "cashed in" after a prescribed period. The policy holder can also borrow against the cash surrender value usually at low interest rates.

Certified Public Accountant (C.P.A.): A title based upon a uniform national examination which acknowledges the competency to practice accounting.

Claims Made Policy: A malpractice insurance policy providing protection only against claims arising within the year the policy is in effect.

Collection Agency: A company who specializes in collecting over-due patient accounts for a fee. The average fee is approximately 50 percent of what is collected.

Collection Percentage: The measurement of the success of a business's efforts to collect for services rendered.

Comprehensive Medical Insurance: A common form of group insurance which provides employees with hospital insurance, surgical insurance, physician expense insurance, and major medical. Many policies require a waiting period before becoming eligible.

Controlling: The managerial function of comparing performance against preset standards and making any necessary corrections.

Corporation: A legal entity authorized by the state to conduct business.

Cost-Benefit Analysis: The process of analyzing an investment to determine whether the future cost savings will justify the purchase decision.

C.P.U.: Central Processing Unit.

Current Assets: Cash and other assets that are expected to be turned into cash or used in the business' normal operating cycle.

Current Liabilities: (Short-term liabilities) Those liabilities that must be paid within the next twelve months.

Day Sheet: A daily record which lists the name of each patient, the amount they were charged, how much was collected, and how much is outstanding.

Deductible: A provision in an insurance policy that requires the policy holder to pay the first $100, $200, $500, or $1,000, before the insurance company will make a payment on a claim.

Defendant: The person or party denying a claim in a lawsuit.

Deposition: Sworn testimony obtained outside of the court room.

Depreciation: An Accounting term reflecting the dollar amount subtracted from an asset due to wear and obselence.

Disbursement Journal: The bookkeeping system of documenting the various amounts of money spent by the practice and on what items and services.

Diskette: A small magnetic disk used for the storage and transfer of data to a computer. Also known as a floppy disk.

Diversification: A practitioner who moves into a totally different line of business.

Economic Analysis: The application of economic theory and methodology to decision making problems in business.

Embezzlement: The appropriation of property or cash through fraud or theft by a person to whom it has been entrusted.

Entrenchment: A marketing term whereby a practitioner responds to increasing competition by attempting to satisfy and retain an established patient market.

Expenses: The costs associated with providing health care.

Expert Witness: An individual requested to provide legal testimony who is recognized as having specialized training, knowledge, or abilities in a given area.

Fact Witness: In health care, an individual who summarizes a treatment provided as well as the patient's response to treatment.

FICA: Federal Insurance Contributions Act. These are taxes paid by both employers and employees. They are commonly known as "Social Security."

Fidelity Bond: An insurance bond written to cover employees who handle financial transactions.

Fixed Assets: An asset such as buildings, land, or equipment which is expected to remain with the practice for an extended period of time.

Fixed Cost: An expense which will not change in the short run regardless of changes in patient volume. Examples include insurance, taxes, and administrative costs.

Generalist: A practitioner who can examine a practice in broad terms and devise methods to alter a practice's direction.

Goodwill: The excess of the selling price over the fair market value of the physical assets.

Group Life Insurance: Usually a fringe benefit offered by the owner of the practice which provides a one-year renewable term policy with the employee paying a portion of the premium. Most policies do not require a physical exam.

Hardware: The computer printer, monitor, keyboard, and other physical equipment needed to run the machines.

Income: Revenue minus expenses. Negative income is defined as a loss.

Income Statement: A financial statement showing the changes which have occurred in the financial performance of the practice over a period of time.

Individual (Sequential) Scheduling: A method of patient scheduling whereby each patient is assigned a specific time for treatment. Patients arrive at the practice at 8:00 a.m., 8:15 a.m., 8:30 a.m., etc.

Influencing: The managerial function of effectively communicating, motivating, and leading personnel to accomplish practice objectives.

Installment Loan: A loan which is repaid gradually over a period of time. Usually on a monthly basis.

Job Descriptions: Job descriptions describe the principle functions and duties of the job as well as the scope of authority.

Job Specifications: A description of the human qualities required for the job including the education, training, experience, and the disposition.

Ledger Card: An individual account receivable which is maintained on each patient showing the charges for services, payments received, and the outstanding balance.

Limited Liability: A feature available to the corporate business community where the shareholder is only liable for the debts of the corporation up to the amount the individual has invested in the corporation. In a professional corporation, the shareholder generally retains their unlimited liability for acts towards patients.

Line Structure: An organizational structure clearly depicting the primary chain of command and line of authority. In every organization there is a direct line of superior/subordinate relationships from the top of the organization to the lowest level of supervision.

Loan Payable: A current installment on a long-term loan which must be paid within the next twelve months.

Long Tail Effect: The requirement that an endorsement be purchased to continue to provide protection under a claims made malpractice insurance policy.

Long Term Liabilities: Those liabilities that are not due and payable within the next twelve months.

Malpractice: An injurous or unprofessional treatment on the part of one engaged in a profession.

Management: The process of accomplishing objectives and goals through people.

Market Development: The attempt by a practitioner to make potential patients aware of the practice. The practitioner is primarily concerned with promoting the practices' present strengths.

Marketing Concepts: Adopting the consumer orientation whereby a practice directs all its efforts at satisfying patients at a profit.

Marketing Mix: The controllable group of variables the practitioner puts together to satisfy the target market.

Medicaid: A government-financed welfare program offering medical assistance to all ages. It is financed partly by each state and partly by the federal government.

Medical Records Release: A document authorizing a practitioner to release copies of patient records only to those individuals as indicated.

Medicare: A program of health insurance established by the federal government primarily for those age sixty-five or older. It covers younger people eligible for disability payments. The program offers two types of insurance; hospital and medical insurance.

Method: Concerned with only one specific step in the performance of a task. The method will describe in writing how one specific step in a task is to be correctly performed.

Microcomputer: Small computers, powered by microchips, which have been designed to be used on desk tops.

Modem: A device that converts data compatible with computer equipment to a form compatible with transmission through telephone lines.

Modified (Rolling Wave) Scheduling: A method of patient scheduling, similar to block scheduling, where each hour is divided into varying treatment times based on rehabilitation requirements.

Monitor (Video Screen): The screen attached to the computer designed for visual display of information.

Net Assets: Total assets minus total liabilities.

Net Income: The excess of revenue over and above expenses during a particular time period. If revenue exceeds expenses, there is a profit. If revenue is less than expenses, there is a loss.

Noncompetition Covenant: A legally enforceable agreement between two or more parties stipulating that individual(s) leaving the practice will not set up a competing practice in the same community.

Occurance Policy: A malpractice insurance policy which protects the therapist against claims arising out of professional actions in a given year regardless of how many years later they will materialize.

Open Door Policy: Management's attempt to openly discuss problems, concerns, or suggestions an employee has about the organization and their individual working environment.

Organizational Chart: Graphically portrays the organization showing the structure, the basic relationships, and grouping of positions and functions.

Organizing: The managerial job of assigning duties and coordinating efforts among practice personnel to ensure objective attainment.

Owners Equity: The share of total assets that remain after the subtraction of the firm's liabilities.

Partnership: An agreement between two or more persons to operate a business as co-owners for a profit.

Patient Charge Ticket: An itemized bill showing the services the patient received.

Petty Cash: A sum of money maintained in an office for the purpose of making small cash purchases.

Planning: The managerial process of setting practice objectives and basic goals and then determining the steps required to attain them.

Plaintiff: The person or party who brings a lawsuit.

Policies: Broad guides to thinking which are designed to aid in channeling the thoughts of personnel charged with decision making.

Prepaid Expenses: An asset representing expenses already paid for in advance that have not been completely used.

Procedures: A guide to employee action, not a guide to thinking. They demonstrate a definite sequence of acts which must be followed to complete a task.

Professional Corporation (Professional Association, Service Corporation): The corporate form of private practice offering advantages in such areas as tax savings and deferral, savings incentives, and employee benefit programs.

Real Estate Option: An agreement between a seller and prospective buyer that states the seller will sell the property to the buyer at a fixed price in the future. In exchange for the right, the prospective buyer gives the seller an agreed upon sum of money.

Revenue: Total charges for services made by the practice during a particular period of time.

Rule: Guides to employee inaction rather than action.

Scalar Structure: The direct line of subordinate/superior relations from the highest level to the lowest managerial positions.

Service Contract: A written agreement which specifies what items will be repaired by a company.

Set Back: A zoning requirement that a structure be built a specified distance from the street.

Severence Pay: The payment and benefit package provided to an employee upon termination.

Single Payment Loan: A loan which is repaid in its entirety on a specific date.

Software: The computer programs used to operate the machine.

Staffing: The managerial function which involves the recruitment, selection, training, compensation, and termination of employees.

Target Market: A fairly similar group of patients to whom a practice wishes to appeal.

Tax Attorney: An attorney who specializes in taxes for individuals and businesses.

Taxes Payable: A current liability owed to the federal, state, or local government.

Term Life Insurance: Provides life insurance protection usually at the lowest premium price. Most term life insurance policies are written for a one-year period.

Unit Scheduling (Patient Grouping): A method of patient scheduling whereby patients are grouped based on treatment similarities or rehabilitation needs.

Unity of Command Principle: A business term indicating every employee should have only one boss. It is management's responsibility to make it apparent to whom each employee will report.

User Friendly: A term common to the computer industry used to describe computers and computer programs which are designed to be easy to understand and use.

Variable Cost: A practice expense that will change in relation to changes in patient volume. As demand increases, these costs will increase. When demand decreases, these expenses will be reduced. An example includes the water requirements for whirlpool therapy.

Whole Life (Ordinary Life) Insurance: An insurance policy which requires the insured to make a series of payments throughout the life of the policy or until he policy is "paid up." The face value is payable upon death.

Word Processing: A computer program designed to aid in producing letter quality documents.

Workers Compensation: A private or state run insurance plan required by law in most states for an employer who has three or more employees. The insurance provides coverage for employment related illness or injury. The employer pays the cost of the insurance.

INDEX